Masculinity and Men's Health

Masculinity and Men's Health

Coronary Heart Disease in Medical and Public Discourse

Elianne Riska

ROWMAN & LITTLEFIELD PUBLISHERS, INC.
Lanham • Boulder • New York • Toronto • Oxford

ROWMAN & LITTLEFIELD PUBLISHERS, INC.

Published in the United States of America
by Rowman & Littlefield Publishers, Inc.
A wholly owned subsidary of The Rowman & Littlefield Publishing Group, Inc.
4501 Forbes Boulevard, Suite 200, Lanham, Maryland 20706
www.rowmanlittlefield.com

PO Box 317
Oxford
OX2 9RU, UK

British Library Cataloguing in Publication Information Available

Library of Congress Cataloging-in-Publication Data

Riska, Elianne.
    Masculinity and men's health : coronary heart disease in medical and public
discourse / Elianne Riska.
        p. cm.
    Includes bibliographical references and index.
    ISBN 0-7425-2900-2 (alk. paper)
    1. Coronary heart disease—Etiology. 2. Type A behavior. 3. Masculinity. I. Title.

    RA645.C68R575 2004
    616.1'23071—dc22   2003069344

Printed in the United States of America

♾™ The paper used in this publication meets the minimum requirements of American
National Standard for Information Sciences—Permanence of Paper for Printed Library
Materials, ANSI/NISO Z39.48-1992.

Contents

Acknowledgments

This book focuses on "Type A," a construct that captured the attention of both physicians and laypeople in the 1960s and early 1970s. The idea was simple and captivating. Its concrete expressions appeared only too visible in the behavior of financial and political leaders: Type A was signified by a certain competitive behavior and personality and seen as a primary reason for men's proneness for coronary heart disease, a major killer in the United States. But what is the standing of this medical concept today—is it valid and useful? There is certainly still a collective memory of Type A as a distinctive behavioral pattern that characterizes competitive, success-oriented, hard-working people. But does this kind of behavior have any bearing on health? The exploration of these questions led to this book.

The origin of this project can be traced back to the 1970s, when I was responsible for introducing students at the College of Human Medicine at Michigan State University to the behavioral aspects of major chronic illnesses. I included among the articles chosen for the curriculum one dealing with Type A that suggested strongly that biomedicine was too narrow a paradigm.

In 1999, in a conversation with David Armstrong in London, Type A came up as an example of the rise and fall of medical ideas. He suggested writing an article about the topic, which eventually appeared in *Social Science and Medicine* in 2000. The key points in that article form the cornerstone of the present book.

Many colleagues have participated in discussions about the topic of this book and have been instrumental in sharpening its theoretical arguments. Among those who have played a crucial role in shaping my sociological thinking on gender are Judith Lorber, Jeff Hearn, and Jan Wickman. Judith Lorber especially elucidated the concept of hardiness. John Wilson brought up the related and relevant concept of John Henryism. Many others have provided helpful comments—for example, Peter Conrad, Barbara Katz-Rothman, Michael Kimmel, Marja-Liisa Honkasalo, Sirpa Wrede, and Dana Rosenfeld.

The writing of the book was facilitated by a yearlong position as a senior researcher in 2002–2003 granted by the Academy of Finland. This leave from teaching at Åbo Akademi University, Finland, allowed the project to be finished within the time planned. A research grant from the Academy of Finland (#200568) enabled the collection of material at American university libraries.

I enjoyed the hospitality of a number of colleagues while I collected the material. Barrie Thorne twice invited me to the University of California, Berkeley, where the early materials on Type A and hardiness were collected. Invitations by Julia McMurray and Myra Marx Ferree to the University of Wisconsin, Madison, enabled research at the libraries on that campus. Invitations by Diane Barthel at the State University of New York, Stony Brook, and by Nicky Hart at the University of California, Los Angeles, similarly enabled me to use the well-supplied libraries on their campuses. I am also grateful to Tom Conner, chair of the Department of Sociology at Michigan State University, who arranged a visit to the department at a crucial point in the writing in the fall of 2002.

A number of colleagues have provided assistance during the final stages of preparing this book for publication. Jeff Hearn read the first full draft of the manuscript, and his comments have much improved its quality. Solveig Bystedt, with her usual patience and kindness, typed the bibliography. And Katherine McCracken has helped me prune the traces of Swedish from my English.

I thank the following journals for giving permission to use and elaborate on previous articles: The Type A man material is reprinted from *Social Science and Medicine*, vol. 51, Elianne Riska, "The Rise and Fall of Type A Man," pp. 1665–1674, copyright © 2000, with permission from Elsevier. The hardy executive material originally appeared as "From Type A Man to the Hardy Man: Masculinity and Health," *Sociology of Health and Illness*, vol. 24, pp. 347–358. The medicalization thesis is reprinted from *Advances in Gender Research*, vol. 7, Elianne Riska, "Gendering the Medicalization Thesis," pp. 61–89, copyright © 2003, with permission from Elsevier.

I am indebted to Dean Birkenkamp, former executive director at Rowman & Littlefield, for his interest in the early outline for a book on Type A and for promoting its realization. I would like to thank Alison Sullenberger, Susan McEachern, Jesse Goodman, Brian Richards, and Alan McClare, who have seen the manuscript through the publication process and into print.

Chapter One

Introduction

In the 1970s the conceptualization of human health in terms of the male as the norm was a common concern among feminist critics of medical knowledge. Among men, this notion did not evoke a broad discussion of the portrayal of their health and body. At the time, there was very little discussion among men that the concept of "man" needed redefinition or demystification. Instead, the biological and "natural" character of men was taken for granted (Hearn 1998). As a consequence, men's health remained gender neutral, a view that rendered the gendered man invisible in most medical research. As Lunbeck notes in her study of American psychiatry from 1900 to 1920 and its view of the modern man, there is a need for research that aims to "tease the gendered man out of the universal Man" (1998, 59). The concept of a universal man has provided a mythic and reductionist picture of men's health by constructing men as a homogeneous group. As a consequence, men's gender and also differences by class and race have tended to be overlooked in past research on men's health.

A look back at the cumulated medical literature on coronary heart disease (CHD), one of the most prevalent health problems during the past fifty years, shows that the studies have taken for granted that they reflect a universal knowledge about human health. A sociological reading of this literature shows that the research contains a variety of etiological theories on *men's* health. These theories harbor a central notion: the health cost of masculinity for white middle-class men. This theme of the middle-class man as victim has had a strong cultural resonance in American society.

Men's health has long been undertheorized by sociologists. By contrast, American psychology began early to address the psychological features of the working man and his health. Through the lens of psychology, American medicine has tried to reach an understanding of the plight of modern men and their health, especially the psychosocial aspects. This trend in etiological thinking began in the 1950s, when the rate of CHD was high for white middle-class men. Since then a number of personality predispositions have been shown to be related to men's risk for developing CHD.

CHD is caused by the hardening of the arteries (atherosclerosis), which are narrowed by fatty deposits. This condition can result in angina (chest pain), heart attack (myocardial infarction), or both. CHD caused 515,204 deaths in the United States in 2000 and is the single leading cause of death in the United States today (American Heart Association 2003).

This book examines the history of those etiological theories proposing that a certain personality predisposition, rather than traditional risk factors (fatty food, smoking, lack of exercise), explains the high CHD mortality rates among American men. Since the 1950s, American psychology has introduced a number of personality types assumed to be related to the prospect of developing CHD. These personality types have been constructed as medical risk factors and have become part of medical discourse. The term *discourse* here means a body of ideas, concepts, and beliefs that have become established as knowledge (e.g., in mainstream medicine) or as an accepted worldview (e.g., public discourse).

This book presents two central arguments about the personality-focused etiological model. The first is that the personality constructs used in medical discourse reflect the cultural representations of masculinity at a given time, but have come to be integrated into medical discourse as reified categories. This book examines three such reified categories: Type A, hardiness, and John Henryism. These personality dispositions, as this book will show, are representations of certain masculinities located in a specific gender, class, and racial order. Each of the personality constructs portrays a certain group of men faced with the effects of structural changes in the contemporary economic and gender orders. As I will show, the constructs harbor notions about the embodied self, social agency, and social structure. Above all, the construction of the three psychological categories not only made visible new dimensions of the health profile of American men, but also became public discourses on the relationship between men's selves, work, and health.

The second argument presented in this book is that the views on masculinity inherent in the medical discourse on men's coronary health have shifted during the past forty years. From a conceptualization of masculine attributes within the framework of sex-role theory making males the victim of a certain social order, the views have moved to an interpretation promoting the masculine subject who can regain autonomy and control over his private and working life and thereby retain his masculinity. In health terms this means that while traditional masculinity was declared a health hazard from the 1950s to the 1970s because of the toll it took on men's health, a slightly refurbished view has since the early 1980s conceptualized the same masculine attributes as promoting health.

There is currently, however, a resurgence of the view of men as victims. Rhetoric about a "crisis of masculinity" is overtly or tacitly appearing in public discourse as media and public policy are pondering the effects of the convergence of gender roles in a time when a large proportion of American women work outside the home. The view of men as victims has been carried over to recent epidemiological thinking. While the men-as-an-endangered-species hypothesis was in the past a metaphor used to portray the crisis experienced by African American men (e.g., Staples 1995b, 136; Dyson 1996, 68), a refurbished version of the hypothesis for the twenty-first century has extended it to include the plight of white middle-class men. For example, the hypothesis has been part of the rhetoric of British public health advocates, who have pointed to men's "health disadvantage." In the fall of 2001, both of the leading British medical journals, *Lancet* (2001) and the *British Medical Journal,* ran editorials on the need to develop the field of men's health. An editorial in the *British Medical Journal* asked for a gender-sensitive approach in future research on CHD, because currently gender is invisible, "resulting in research that does not consider the issue of masculinity and men's acknowledged difficulty in managing their health" (White and Lockyer 2001, 1016). Another editorial posed the provocative question, "Are men in danger of extinction?" and pondered, "Are there effective and morally acceptable strategies to modify men's negative behaviour towards themselves and others" (Meryn and Jadad 2001, 1013).

In the spring of 2003 the *American Journal of Public Health* published a special issue on men's health. The editorials remarked that "the subject of men's health is frequently neglected in public health discussions" (Meyer 2003, 709) and that "poor men had become invisible and their health needs neglected" (Treadwell and Ro 2003; see also Williams 2003).

The new public health interest in men's health—called men's health discourse—rests on the assumption that "men suffer a health disadvantage that is comparable to, if not greater than women's" (Schofield et al., 2000, 248). As many critics have noted, such a view of men as victims promotes a picture of a mythical, homogeneous group of men (Brittan 1989; Whitehead 2002). It is therefore important to take this picture apart and, thereby, promote a broader sociological understanding that not only deconstructs the homogeneous notion of men and masculinity by pointing to diversity by class, race, and sexual orientation, but also traces the emergence of the victimhood of men and analyzes the notion of the health costs for men of such a victimhood.

There is a growing body of American and British scholarship that examines changing definitions of masculinity and how conceptions of masculinity are part of institutions and economic structures (e.g., Hearn 1996 and 1998; Kimmel 2000). This scholarship, as British sociologist Petersen bemoans, contains few histories that "focus explicitly and systematically on the frameworks of knowledge within which 'masculinity' and the male subject have been constructed" (1998, 9).

This book looks at how medicine has constructed masculinity and masculine behavior as medical categories. The book employs a key construct in post–World War II American medicine—Type A—to illustrate the gendered character of men's health and the changes in the focus of victimization theory as it relates to men. A certain cultural repertoire of men's emotions—anger, aggression, competitiveness—was medicalized by a new psychosocial discourse in medicine that began to explore men's interiors as the reason for their propensity to develop CHD.

It is important to be aware of the cultural dimension of the Type A phenomenon. The rise of Type A is a time-bound and cultural concept. Type A came to resonate with the way that Americans interpreted the characteristics needed for success in white-collar work and the personal costs for such material endeavors. While writing this book I came, in an anecdotal way, to experience the impact of the concept of Type A on public imagery in the United States. When middle-aged Americans—academic or nonacademic, male or female—learned that I was writing a book about Type A, I was astounded to find how vivid the collective memory of this concept was. People began spontaneously to reminiscence and discuss it. By contrast, in the European context, almost without exception, my mentioning the theme of my book drew blank stares, or even bewilderment, because the concept has been totally absent from public discourse in Europe. I soon realized that Type A was a uniquely American collective image.

Type A is shown to be a culture-bound phenomenon, the utility of which was restricted by time, place, gender, race, and social class. Nevertheless, it became a core concept in American medicine after World War II and provided a powerful cultural image for understanding the cause of the medical risk of men's developing CHD. At the same time it pointed to the crisis of the self-made man in the American economy and its gender system. Underlying the concept was the need to understand the health consequences for white middle-class men of the rapid change in the U.S. economy and gender system. Type A became part of American folklore and a common tale of work behavior, a tale that valorized, but also hesitantly began to deplore, such behavior. But the discourse on Type A became, too, a tale that translated commonsense knowledge of men's work behavior into naturalized notions of personality. I will show that medicine absorbed a cultural representation of masculinity at a specific historical moment and cultural setting in American society and constructed this representation as a medical and psychological fact, which was then embodied as a material practice. In this regard, medicine constructed, but also challenged, conventional knowledge of "male nature." The historical production of this medical knowledge is the central theme of this book.

This volume argues that the personality-focused etiological theories of CHD promote an individualistic approach to illness, an approach that will here be called *psychologism*. Explanations that take as their departure the idea that social phenomena can be reduced to psychological phenomena adopt this approach (Popper 1962, 88–98). This type of explanation, furthermore, is based on *methodological individualism,* which takes its departure from the assumption that the behavior and attitudes of social groups can be reduced to the behavior and the actions of individuals (Popper 1962, 91). Collective or social phenomena are, according to this view, merely the aggregate of the actions and attitudes of single individuals, rather than reflections of shared material conditions, experiences of the social environment, or effects of a social institution.

STRUCTURE OF THE BOOK

This book focuses on the rise of one health agenda in the late 1950s for the white middle-class American man and its consequences not only for how men's health has later been conceptualized, but also how health research in general has been pursued. The medical discourse on Type A captured the crisis and the cultural critique of key middle-class values in the mid-1950s, issues that later became the focus of a number of middle-class movements — the student movement, the new women's movement, the consumer movement — in the mid-1960s. But the medical discourse on Type A preceded these movements by almost a decade. This discourse became a tacit critique of the moral ambiguity of the dominant form of white middle-class masculinity. It pointed out the health hazards of overconformity to what Kimmel has called a "blind pursuit of a marketplace masculinity" and of the antisocial and self-destructive character of the self-made man (1997, 266).

Chapter 2 suggests that a notion of victimhood underlies most etiological thinking on men's health. It presents a review of the basic assumptions surrounding the notion of the victimized male with a description of the assumed impact of this status on men's health. The chapter examines the medicalization thesis and the invisibility of men's health within this framework of the analysis of gender and health.

Chapter 2 then reviews the book's methodological approach. In the analysis of the topic, a Foucauldian "genealogical method" is used (Armstrong 1990; Foucault 1975), the purpose of which is to trace the origin of three psychological categories: Type A personality, hardiness, and John Henryism. The task is to unfold the historical epistemology of these psychological categories (Rose 1999; Danziger 1997; Aronowitz 1998). The construction of these three categories reveals new dimensions of the health profile of American men.

The data were gathered through an examination of pioneering scientific articles and the subsequent use of the constructs. The analysis reported is qualitative. It examines the scientific discovery of a certain type of personality assumed to explain the prevalence of CHD among American men. In focus are the methods and data sections of the scientific articles, which describe the subjects of the research and the construction of the instruments. The development of new psychological tests enabled the mapping of the phenomenon. The instruments (i.e., the scales developed) have produced and confirmed the psychological categories constructed in this way.

Chapter 3 shows how the concept of Type A became the subject of a new medical discourse that in the late 1950s revealed the "cause" of CHD. The Type A man, characterized by Type A behavioral pattern, or TABP, became visible through a new medical gaze. The emergence of this social and diagnostic category was tied to the medicalization of the attributes of traditional white middle-class masculinity. The Type A discourse resonated with the kind of normative masculinity and the kind of challenges the male breadwinner ideal encountered as a consequence of the Great Depression and after the end of World War II.

Chapter 3 documents the social construction of Type A man in the American scientific medical literature in the 1950s and 1960s. The data include medical articles published on the topic of Type A from 1955 onward. The chapter traces how Type A was originally defined and what kinds of instruments were used to measure the Type A behavioral pattern. It also looks at the character of Type B and Type C men as they were described in the original model, as well as at the portrayal of the "health hazard" for Type A and Type B men of a working spouse and how this hazard was described in the early Framingham Heart Study.

Chapter 4 argues that the Type A concept lost its utility when the construct was taken over by the psychologists, whose efforts to measure the psychological dimensions of the "coronary-prone personality" and behavioral pattern eventually fragmented the concept. The Type A behavioral pattern, which characterized Type A, could no longer be used by the doctors as a simple behavioral indicator of a man's risk of heart disease. The psychological concept—the coronary-prone personality, or the Type A personality—was further developed in health psychology and stress research.

Chapter 5 describes the transition in American research from the focus on Type A man to that of the hardy man in the early 1980s. These two diagnostic categories were constructed in medical and psychological discourse and entailed certain notions of masculinity, class, and health. While Type A had been a construct that explained the rise of unhealthy (coronary-prone) American middle-class white men in the 1950s, the construct of the hardy executive explained the existence of healthy and hardy men in the same class, race, and gender order in the late 1970s. The chapter shows that the construction of Type A man rested on the medicalization of the core values of traditional masculinity, while the new term *hardy man* demedicalized and legitimized these values.

Chapter 5 uses Foucault's notion of technologies of the self to indicate how hardiness is a quality expected of the successful middle-class male executive. The concept of the hardy man offers a method for mastery and development of the self. Hardiness is the kind of self-discipline expected of economic actors who work in an economy and labor market characterized by flexibility and short-term jobs. The hardy executive construct points to the resurrection of the moral dimension—men of character—of current capitalism, a moral foundation thought lost in a post-Fordist economy (e.g., Sennett 1998). The hardy man construct also restored the masculine subject, a perception of a man as one who has recaptured his agency. The construct provides a legitimation for dominant masculinity by restoring the key values of modern masculinity. This construct can therefore be seen as a response to the need to act on the crisis of masculinity. This argument will be further illuminated by looking back at the roots of the cultural production of the hardy male in American popular culture.

Chapter 6 examines the kind of personality constructed to incorporate the hard-working African American man into the model. A new construct, John Henryism, was introduced in the literature on cardiovascular disease in the early 1980s. This is a personality predisposition that is assumed to make African American men prone to hypertension. The chapter argues that the construct of John Henryism rests on a cultural representation of the so-called race man (Drake and Cayton 1945, 394–395; Carby 1998), a racialized construction of man. The research on John Henryism has shown that it is associated with high blood pressure and hypertension—major risk factors for CHD—among African American men.

Chapter 7 examines the medical thinking that locates the reason for men's high CHD rates in their personalities. Nevertheless, the personal attributes described were not really individual ones because they captured the cultural features of a certain revered type of masculinity. This cultural representation of masculinity has been reified in medicine and comes to be treated as a major medical risk factor. Chapter 7 presents the constructive scheme for the devel-

opment of the measurement techniques for mapping the type of personality believed to constitute the major risk factor for developing CHD. The techniques
for the production of the major constructs are examined: Type A, Type B, hardiness, and John Henryism.

Chapter 8 identifies the social categories of men introduced in the CHD
literature—Type A, the hardy executive, the John Henry man—and their location in the prevailing gender, economic, and racial order. The chapter presents a comparison of the assumed behavioral and attitudinal characteristics of
the Type A, the hardy executive, and the John Henry man and the types of
masculinity they represent. The views of Robert Merton, C. Wright Mills, and
Richard Sennett illuminate the relationship between character and social
structure. The chapter argues that the agentic character of men and the crisis
of masculinity are notions hidden in the etiological theories on CHD.

The concluding chapter explores why the concept of Type A has survived
so long in American public discourse after its demise in medicine. There is a
paradox in the public discourse in that, today, Type A is used to indicate the
kind of lifestyle that is bad for physical and mental health, regardless of gender. Still, Type A remains an idiom in working life. The work behavior and
ethic of Type A man is the norm against which commitment to and behavior
at work are evaluated. Increasingly, new technologies of the self that valorize
self-management and self-discipline are promoted in working life so as to
make those people who are committed to the values of work more fit for current organizational work arrangements. The hardy man is still the model of
self that seems most fit to carry out the mission of the new culture and social
order of a post-Fordist economy.

New therapeutic approaches have emerged that purport to address the
"space of anxiety," a discourse that interprets mental health problems as related to the private self, rather than reflecting the structural arrangement of
work (Young 1980; Rose 1999). The most recent personality construct in the
alphabet is Type D, which stands for the "distressed" personality (Denollet
2000; Denollet and Van Heck 2001; Denollet et al., 1995 and 1996). Type D
has been presented as an independent risk factor for cardiac problems in patients with documented CHD.

The central argument of this book is that a gender-neutral approach to
work-related stress and distress misses the rich scientific history of medical
research and the past fifty years' etiological thinking on men's major chronic
disease—CHD. A sociological reading of this scientific literature uncovers its
gendered notions. While the aim of the personality-focused etiological theories of CHD has been to find a universal explanation for the emergence of
heart disease, the constructs—the personalities—have been culture bound
and male gendered. The analysis points to the social construction of medical

and psychological categories in medical knowledge. This medical knowledge has tacitly highlighted the masculine, but treated it as universal, rather than male gendered, and thereby rendered both the gendered character of men's health and women's heart disease invisible. Chapter 9 concludes with the observation that health research is not for one gender only and that future research and theorizing on health needs to take a gender-informed approach.

Chapter Two

The Victimized Self: Men's Personality as a Medical Risk Factor

The subject of gender and health is still understood by many to refer to "women's health" because women's health became a concern of feminist activists in the 1970s. In the 1980s and 1990s the demand for new knowledge in the field generated both new empirical knowledge and theoretical frameworks for understanding women's health from a gender perspective (see Lorber and Moore 2002; Annandale and Hunt 2000). This research has shown that women report psychological and somatic symptoms far more often than men do and that women also report chronic illness more often. Public health advocates remain concerned, however, that men still have a higher mortality rate than women. While women more often than men report health problems or a chronic illness, men in the Western world tend to live five to seven years less than women. This phenomenon has been captured in a catchy and illuminating saying: "Women get sicker, but men die quicker" (Lorber and Moore 2002, 13). Furthermore, over the past thirty years, health researchers and health promoters in most Western countries have documented that men use health services less than women do, and it has been argued that men underutilize these services.

There is a paradox in these figures and in the related interpretations of the gender differential in the use of health services. In the 1970s, feminists criticized women's frequent use of health care and suggested that their rate of use amounted to overutilization. This overutilization, it was argued, was prompted by a male-dominated medical profession and a profit-seeking drug industry, which medicalized women's "normal" symptoms and everyday life events and, thereby, increased women's presumed need for treatment. They assumed that these practices arose out of a sexist ideology, one that interpreted a woman's body as pathological and her mind as emotional and passive because the male body and the "rational" mind of men were used as the

11

single and universal standard of human health (e.g., Chesler 1989, 69; see also Eichler 1980). Broverman and her colleagues documented this "double standard of health" in a study on American clinicians' views about what kind of behavioral traits were healthy in an adult (1970). The study showed that clinicians' conceptions of healthy mature men did not differ significantly from their conceptions of healthy adults. Furthermore, clinicians were less likely to attribute traits associated with healthy adults to a woman than to a man (Broverman et al., 1970, 5). The study concluded that the general standard of health is applied only to men, while healthy women are perceived as significantly less healthy by adult standards. These findings confirm the notion of the "unmarked" character of male bodies (see Robinson 2000, 1). Men's bodies are seen as unmarked and disembodied of male gender, and their bodies and health come therefore to represent the universal and the generic standard of human health. This disembodied universality of men's health stands in sharp contrast to the marked and embodied character of women's bodies (and the bodies of racial groups other than Caucasians).

Nevertheless, the female and not the male standard has been used by public health advocates as the statistical norm for a proper use of health services. This normative muster has meant that men's underutilization has been constructed by taking women's usage of health services as the universal norm. Still, when men's rates approach women's rates of illnesses or use of services, this phenomenon is interpreted as a departure from the masculine norm and as men's "health disadvantage." In his comments on the Australian debate, Connell (2000, 193) proposes that the crisis in men's health seems exaggerated since men as a group have rates of illness similar to or lower than women's. For him, the crisis rhetoric feeds a general victimization thinking about men's social position. In this regard, figures on men's mortality and health disadvantage have been used as emblematic of a much broader and serious cultural phenomenon: men are identified as the new "disadvantaged" (Whitehead 2002, 51). The argument seems tautological because the crisis of masculinity seems to be both the cause for the disadvantage's emergence and the reason for its prevalence. But as Whitehead (2002, 59) has suggested, the crisis-of-masculinity discourse reveals the importance of understanding men and masculinity as discursive and the need to unravel the culture-specific claims of such argumentation.

THE VICTIMIZED MALE AND HIS HEALTH

The gender identity and gender division of labor between men and women were given a social-scientific explanation in the late 1930s when sex-role

theory was introduced. Over the next thirty years, this theory became a powerful framework for interpreting the sex-role identities and functions of men
and women in the family (Pleck 1981; Messner 1998). Women social scientists were the first to assess the sex-role theory critically. In the 1970s, feminist critics began to interpret sex-role theory as an ideology of the nuclear
family and as a tacit legitimation of the dominance of men over women. Nevertheless, it is important to remember that at its inception sex-role theory was
not a conservative framework. On the contrary, the theory offered a sociological view that departed from and radically challenged the prevailing biological view of male and female nature. By locating the sex roles in values
and institutions, sex-role theory offered a potential for change rather than taking biology as destiny. The conservative climate of the 1950s confirmed,
however, the traditional sex roles of the nuclear family as a sound societal
structure. The advocates of sex-role theory tended to demand that individuals
fit these roles rather than that the roles change in order to fit the diversity of
individuals. The latter issue became the theme of the criticism of the women's
movement of the 1960s.

Sex-role theory has been a major paradigm for understanding male identity
in scientific and public discourse (Pleck 1981; Messner 1998). The paradigm
set the parameters of the normal psychological and social development of the
American boy and man and in this way defined a kind of prototype of
"healthy sex-role identity" for males (Pleck 1981, 3; Brittan 1989, 26). A
strong male sex-role identity has been equated with a healthy male identity.

As critical reviewers of sex-role theory have noted, this theoretical framework does not identify any problems as related to the sex roles as such, but
rather to individuals unable to fit the script. For the critics, the reference to
the functionality of the sex roles as a reason for their existence is tautological
and, hence, not a satisfactory explanation for their origin and existence. Thus,
the theory can explain why people adopt the appropriate sex role, but it can
neither explain why or how the script has been institutionalized, nor account
for changes, either at the individual or the social level (Pleck 1981; Brittan
1989; Walby 1990; Messner 1998; Kimmel 2000).

The rise of the men's liberation movement in the 1970s resulted in a criticism of the traditional male role and the narrow and limiting character of this
role for men. Nevertheless, at the same time there emerged a movement
among other men to restore and revitalize the values and behaviors of traditional masculinity (Messner 1998; Kimmel and Kaufman 1995). It is therefore important to distinguish, as Pleck does in his path-breaking review of
two types of male role: the *traditional* and the *modern* (1976, 156–157). The
traditional male role is validated through display of physical strength, and
anger and impulsive behavior are encouraged, especially with other males,

while interpersonal and emotional skills are prohibited. The modern version of the male role, Pleck argues, privileges interpersonal skills and an emotionally constrained self.

Taking the traditional and modern male roles as reference points, Pleck identifies two major perspectives in defining the strains and problems in men's roles: the sex-role-identity perspective identifies the problem as lying in men's sex-role identity; the sex-role-strain perspective defines the problem as a strain in the expectations and demands of the traditional and modern male roles. The sex-role-identity perspective identifies traditional masculinity and its related behaviors and traits as desirable, even as imperative for the "normal" and "healthy" development of a boy and man. It is assumed that modern society does not provide boys with concrete male role models in the family or school and that boys and men do not have access to activities and experiences that offer them opportunities to validate their masculinity and maleness. The sex-role-strain perspective suggests that men have been socialized in traditional values, but are expected to behave like modern men, or that the modern male role still is too narrow and conflicts with the assumed universal human need for intimacy (Pleck 1976, 158–159).

The two perspectives on the problems of the male sex role appear also in the literature examining the cultural features of men's health. Studies have pointed to the lethal character of traditional masculinity and the health costs of the traditional and modern male roles (e.g., Harrison et al., 1989; Helgeson 1995; Sabo and Gordon 1995; Messner 1997; Courtenay 2000). This literature has brought to the surface what will here be called the victimization view of men's health.

The victimization argument is represented by two interpretations. The first interpretation, based on a sex-role-identity perspective, suggests that the operative effects of the male mystique—men's self-destructive and risky behavior engaged in to prove traditional masculinity and heterosexual male identity—influence men's life expectancy. This "dark side" of masculinity (Brooks 2001, 287) is a leading cause of death among younger men (homicide, reckless driving, drinking, drug-taking). Such a notion of the male victim has been the rallying cry of a rightist men's movement in the United States (Kimmel and Kaufman 1995). The men's rights discourse has portrayed men as the true victims of the current gender system, which has enabled women's liberation, but kept men in their traditional role as primary breadwinners. This rightist discourse has focused on the "victimized male" and privileged the resurrection of an essentialist masculine identity—a "deep, essential manhood"—that is seen as equivalent to a healthy masculinity (Kimmel and Kaufman 1995, 21; Nonn 1995, 174; Messner 1998, 266).

The second interpretation of the health costs of traditional masculinity is based on the sex-role-strain perspective. It suggests that the current gender system assigns men primary economic responsibility, which constrains modern men to live fully up to their human potential. This interpretation is represented by the liberal strand of the men's movement, which criticizes the traditional male role as oppressive. Modern men want to change, but they are trapped in a narrow economic role in the public sphere and with few opportunities for human growth and for participating in the care of their children. This view has been called the "discourse on male inexpressivity" (Robinson 2002, 208). Men become emotionally blocked and crippled because they are caught in the rat race of economic success. Critics of the liberal view of men's liberation have pointed to the essentialist notion inherent in the "blockage-release model" of men's physical and emotional energies (Robinson 2002, 225). This model harbors essentialist conceptions of masculinity, a masculinity that on the one hand is wounded by any blockage, but on the other seems to be untempered by change.

The liberal strand of the men's movement in the 1970s was committed to a belief in gender symmetry. The assumption here is that traditional sex roles hurt both men and women more or less equally. While women are "sex objects," men are "success objects" trapped in the structuring of the labor market (McMahon 1993, 689; Messner 1998, 261). This view of gender as conformity (Connell 2000, 7) is interpreted against the backdrop of a sexist consumer culture assumed to commodify and objectify both the female and the male. The remedy seems to be for men and women to unite against the common enemy—the consumerist culture. The consumerist culture is seen as having tarnished a more "pure" androgynous category of the two genders. What this strand of thinking results in is a homogenization and naturalization of the kind of ideal versions of gender it promotes. But, above all, this view does not take into account the institutionalized system of unequal power that underlies the prevailing gender system. Instead the gender system is seen as based on certain values and a common culture that can be redefined and fought against only if it is properly identified and declared undesirable.

The victimization view of masculinity is today tied to the claim of a crisis in men's health and the concomitant claim of men's health disadvantage. Recently, four critical observations have been made to counter this kind of conceptualization and claim. First, the claim rests on a notion of a homogeneous body of men in crisis (Brittan 1989, 183). As R. W. Connell observes, if there ever was a men's health crisis, it was in the 1960s, when heart disease was high among post–World War II men (2000, 193). As many critics have noted, men are not a homogeneous group, but differentiated by class, race, and sexual orientation. In this regard, the health crisis currently concerns only very specific groups of men—that is, men marginalized by race and social class (e.g., Whitehead 2002, 54; Connell 2000; Courtenay and Keeling 2000; Schofield et al., 2000).

Second, the claim of a crisis in men's health is based on an ahistorical notion of a static and universal standard of men's health. The myth of masculinity as the disembodied norm has rendered invisible the dominance of white men both in representation and in the realm of the social. The unmarked character of men—for example, men's body and health as the generic category—has had its own logic, according to feminist critics of the men's health question (e.g., Robinson 2000; Davis 2002). Making the normative visible as a category in embodied and racialized terms would call into question the privileges of unmarkedness that men currently enjoy (Hearn 1998; Robinson 2000, 1–3; Davis 2002, 58).

Third, there is an underlying view of gender parity. The assumption is that men and women in the twenty-first century share a mutual suffering and health disadvantage because the new gender equality has generated a convergence of gender roles in the sphere of work and the family (Messner 1998; Schofield et al., 2000, 248). The assumption is that women's liberation and more recent labor-market participation have improved the quality of life of women, but created a new disadvantage for men. It is true that research in the Western world shows that when women enter the labor market, their health improves rather than deteriorates. Nevertheless, this kind of interpretation of women's health does not look closely at the segregations of labor along traditional gender lines in both the public and the private spheres or at the health impact these—called the first and second shift, respectively (Hochschild 1997)—will have on women's health in the long run.

Fourth, the rhetoric of the men's health disadvantage and men's health crisis, according to British observers (e.g., Brittan 1989, 181–194; Connell 2000, 195; Whitehead 2002, 51), has to be seen as a form of backlash against women and feminism. According to Brittan (1989, 184), underlying the crisis-of-masculinity thesis is a "legitimation crisis": male authority can no longer be taken for granted. But the crisis rhetoric does not have to mean a destabilization of the dominant groups of men (Brittan 1989, 186; Hearn 1996). In the American context, Sally Robinson points to the emergence of an identity politics of the dominant, in which the victimization of the white male plays a significant part (2000, 11–12, and 2002, 207). Men, in contrast to women, lack a concrete oppressor and enemy, and so men construct themselves as wounded by their own power, by responsibility, and by the gender order itself. As Robinson suggests, "Representations of wounded white men most often work to personalize the crisis of white masculinity and, thus, to erase the personal and political causes and effects" (2000, 8). She suggests that the rhetoric of crisis and the victimization view—claiming the status of wounded—serve the purpose of reimagining and thereby confirming the dominant meanings of white masculinity.

In short, the argument of the "burden" of the breadwinner male role and the notion of the "victimized" (Nonn 1995) and "wounded" (Robinson 2000 and

2002) male do not view the male role through the lens of the economic and social privilege enjoyed by men in the prevailing economic and gender system. The belief that men are more seriously victimized than women renders invisible the health-promoting aspects of men's privileged position within existing race, class, and gendered hierarchies and men's access to and control over valuable resources (Messner 1998; Doyal 2001, 1062; Schofield et al., 2000). As several critics have pointed out (Connell 1995; Kimmel 2000, 89), sex-role theory treats gender as a role, rather than as a social position with invested power. More importantly, sex-role theory makes invisible the gender system as an institution based on men's power of superordination and on inequality between the sexes. As Hearn suggests, "Deconstructing the dominant (or the superordinate) involves making clearer the social construction of 'men,' 'whiteness,' of 'able-bodiedness' and so on" (1996, 614).

In the past, the image of themselves as victims of traditional sex roles has not had as powerful an appeal to men as it had to women in mobilizing them to advocate for more research and health policy measures to improve their health. For women, the sex-role theory of women's health pointed to health disadvantages for all women. Feminists pointed to the cultural hegemony of medicine, to the male domination among physicians, and to the loss of power of women as consumers of health care. The view of medicine as a gendered organization and male-dominated culture has therefore been powerful gender imagery for women, one that made all women the victims of a gender ideology assumed to permeate medicine as a body of knowledge and as a health care system. This imagery made visible the institutionalized gender and power structure influencing the kind of health care women tend to receive, especially in the areas of reproductive and mental health (Boston Women's Health Collective 1973).

A collective image of men as disadvantaged has so far not been able to mobilize men for a common cause to advance their health needs. As some scholars have suggested, in a culture that valorizes agency, power, and control as the norm of masculinity, men would transgress the norm of a unified masculinity by admitting a position of disadvantage and powerlessness (Davis 2002, 60). Nevertheless, the victimization view is hidden in etiological theories on diseases specific to men—for example, CHD.

VICTIMIZATION THEORY AND MEDICALIZATION OF THE RISKS OF THE HEART DISEASE VICTIM

The metaphor of men as victims is by definition one that points to men's blocked agency. The sociological term *agency* means here that human beings are perceived as having the capacity to influence events and to behave to some extent independently of the constraints of society (e.g., Giddens 1986, 14). The kind of personality theories constructed in the scientific discourse of psychology have emphasized men's agency as their natural status and healthy identity. American psychological discourse has constructed men's agency as that of a rational autonomous subject for whom it is natural to exert control and power. In my analysis, victimization is a sense of a wounded self (see also Wainwright and Calnan 2002, 156; Robinson 2002, 225). Nevertheless, both the pathologized and the normal self are related to the cultural and social context. As Kai Erikson suggests in his classic work on the topic, "The deviant and the conformist, then, are creatures of the same culture, inventions of the same imagination" (1966, 21).

I argue here that the experience of a wounded self is gendered and related to men's situation in the gender order as experienced against the backdrop of a binary gender order in which women are subordinate to men (Lorber 2000). Men occupy a social position of superordination vis-à-vis women as a group, a social position that maximizes men's agency. Restricted agency results in the pathologization of the experience of any limitations in fulfilling the active self, an experience not gender neutral, but related to a man's lived experience of selfhood. The experiences are also lived within the framework of a hierarchical gender order such that a certain group of men—white heterosexual middle-class men—exert cultural, social, and economic power over other men (Connell 1987). The victimization view as applied to health is therefore a gendered theory, and in the field of men's health, it rests on men's embodied experience of masculinity. As Whitehead has defined embodied masculinity,

> Masculine bodily existence suggests the occupation of space, the capacity to define space, the ability to exercise control over space and a preparedness to put one's body at risk in order to achieve these expectations. The male/boy/man is *expected* to transcend space, or to place his body in aggressive motion within it, in so doing posturing to self and others the assuredness of his masculinity. (2002, 189)

The following chapters show how in the twentieth century the CHD literature has medicalized men's agency, especially with reference to a man's capacity to control his inner self and his external environment. They demonstrate that explanations of men's propensity for developing heart disease medicalized a number of values and behaviors that were crucial parts of white middle-class masculinity in the 1950s and 1960s. For example, a certain kind of aggressive and competitive (male) conduct—the Type A personality—became a risk factor for CHD. This explanation captured men's emotional "nature" by heralding the inner self as the core of the essential man, but also by constructing men's emotional being as their personalities. The medical discourse on Type A pathologized men's cultural repertoire of violent emotions—anger, hostility, and aggressiveness.

In the 1970s, the medicalization thesis became an analytical tool for feminist critics in understanding how medicine as a cultural system tended to reinforce women's traditional sex roles. Women began to challenge the traditional roles assigned to them by society at large by organizing into a new wave of the feminist movement and the women's health movement (Ruzek 1978). For men such initiatives for reforming men's roles remained largely marginal (Messner 1998). Instead, medicine and psychology channeled the signals of strains and pressures in men's traditional roles and integrated them into scientific discourse. Such discourse portrayed men as unmarked by gender, class, and race. This meant that the unmarked bodies and minds of men were integrated into the scientific discourse of medicine and psychology as the natural categories of Type A and Type A personality.

At the same time a broader shift in the etiology of chronic illnesses took place. The risk-factor approach emerged from a new multicausal medical thinking that integrated psychological factors into the new epidemiology. A new term *psychosocial factors* was later added to the vocabulary of the risk-factor approach. A psychosocial factor has been defined as "a measurement that potentially relates psychological phenomena to the social environment and to pathophysiological changes" (Hemingway and Marmot 1999, 1460). The risk-factor approach pointed to specific, quantifiable, and manageable mechanisms and paradoxically resulted, as the next section shows, in reductionist thinking about the etiology of heart disease (Aronowitz 1998).

THE MEDICALIZATION THESIS

The medicalization thesis derives from a classic theme in the field of medical sociology. It addresses the broader issue of the power of medicine—as a culture and as a profession—to define and regulate social behavior. This issue was introduced into sociology fifty years ago by Talcott Parsons, who suggested that medicine was a social institution that regulated the kind of deviance for which the individual was not held morally responsible and for which a medical diagnosis could be found (1951). The agent of social control was the medical profession, an institutionalized structure that had been given the mandate to restore the sick to health so that they could resume their expected role obligations. Inherent to this view of medicine was the functionalist perspective on the workings of society: the basic function of medicine was to maintain the established social division of labor, a state that guaranteed the optimum working of society. For twenty years, the Parsonian interpretation of how medicine worked—including sick-role theory and the theory of the profession of medicine—constituted the mainstream of the bourgeoning field of medical sociology.

Thirty years ago, when Irving Zola introduced the notion of medicine as an institution of social control, it was not therefore a totally new way of thinking (1972). The medicalization thesis addresses the normative and control function of medicine, a notion central to Parsons's view of medicine (1951). The medicalization thesis has been developed further by Zola's students, among whom Peter Conrad has been its most eminent interpreter. According to Conrad, the term *medicalization* denotes a process by which nonmedical problems are defined and treated as medical problems, usually as illnesses or disorders (1992, 209): "Medicalization consists of defining a problem in medical terms, using medical language to describe a problem, adopting a medical framework to understand a problem, or using a medical intervention to 'treat it'" (Conrad 1992, 211, and 2000, 322).

The sociologically innovative contribution of the medicalization thesis was the challenge that medicine was delegated a task and power that extended its original mandate. Zola did not see this process as an imperialistic act of the medical profession alone, but rather, as he phrased it, as "an insidious and often undramatic phenomenon accomplished by 'medicalizing' much of daily living, by making medicine and the labels 'healthy' and 'ill' relevant to an ever increasing part of human existence" (Zola 1972, 487). The reason for the "medicalizing of society process" was, according to Zola, the increasingly complex technological and bureaucratic system that fed a reliance on the expert (1972, 496, 487). Even in this sense the involvement of medical expertise in the management of society was hardly novel since public health, preventive medicine, and psychiatry had been given a built-in social emphasis and the task of regulating human behavior (Zola 1972, 488).

"The medicalizing of society," as Zola called it, later became known as the medicalization thesis (1972). The vulgar version of this thesis has tended to identify the medical profession as a promoter of medical imperialism and the patient as the victim of medicine's professional and economic desire to retain professional control over phenomena related to health. For Zola, medicalization seemed more to be propelled by a cultural climate that looks for technical solutions to essentially social problems than merely to be the product of the desire of the medical profession to extend its professional domain. In Zola's analysis, medicalization is a tendency to reduce a social problem to an individual one and to find a technical—in other words, medical—solution at the individual level. As Zola puts it, "By locating the source and the treatment of problems in an individual, other levels of intervention are effectively closed" (Zola 1972, 500). For those familiar with C. Wright Mills's (1959, 8) analysis of society, the process that Zola refers to is the tendency to turn public issues of social structure into personal troubles of milieu.

As Zola suggested in his pioneering essay, medicalization was propelled by a change in the medical thinking from a specific etiology to a multicausal one, one suggesting that it is necessary to intervene to change the habits of a patient's lifetime (1972, 493). Behavioral medicine has focused on the behavioral components of illness and how cultural and psychological factors influence certain kinds of behavior that are detrimental or beneficial to a person's health. The behavioral and psychosocial factors became the new aspects of health and illness, aspects that had not previously been seen as part of the jurisdiction of medicine. Preventive medicine became an essential part of this new medical thinking. This field of medicine has its roots in the risk-factor approach, especially as related to CHD. As Aronowitz has suggested, when mortality and morbidity from acute infectious diseases declined, the rates of chronic diseases began to increase (1998, 122). This "epidemiological transition" changed the medical thinking about and prognoses of diseases and shifted the focus to specific and preventable individual risk factors. Conrad has called this aspect "healthicization," a trend characterized by the advancement of behavioral and social definitions for previously biomedically defined events—for example, heart disease (1992, 223). While medicalization denotes a process whereby the moral turns into the medical, healthicization connotes a process whereby health turns into the moral—for example, the obligation to adopt a healthy lifestyle. According to Aronowitz, "risk factors thus gave scientific backing for timeless and appealing notions that link individual choice and responsibility with health and disease" (1998, 138).

Healthy-lifestyle thinking has been represented by a larger cultural trend in society that Crawford has called "healthism" (1980). This concern with personal health and self-care endeavors is a lay effort to improve personal health. Crawford interprets such efforts within a larger sociopolitical system that does not initiate larger political changes that would influence health. In addition to this power perspective, there is the neoliberal interpretation promoted by those sociologists who perceive identity as tied to a "reflexive project of the self" and part of the emergence of a posttraditional social order (e.g., Giddens 1991). According to this view, reflexive modernity provides the context for a lifestyle discourse of the self and self-help, and the culture of healthism becomes part of exploring and constructing the self.

Over the past thirty years, the medicalization thesis has been a way of interpreting the reasons behind the expansion of high-tech medicine and preventive medicine. The thesis contains a criticism of this development as not promoting health, but rather certain vested interests. The view is that medical science and medical technology have their own imperative as driving forces in shaping health care (e.g., Timmermans and Berg 2003, 99). The orthodox notion of the thesis interprets patients as medicalized victims of the power of medicine. Critics have suggested that it is an illusion that health care could be totally demedicalized (Lupton 1997, see also Riessman 1992). They argue that the existence of a pure nonmedicalized knowledge is hardly possible in Western societies. Representatives of a Foucauldian approach, who suggest that medicine is a disciplinary regime, have proposed this view. This Foucauldian interpretation defines individuals as actors, but also as actors who have internalized the message of self-discipline and self-control inherent in the healthy-lifestyle theory and its message of health promotion. It is in this sense that self-help, self-care, and psychological theories about self-advancement and increase of self-control in working and private life have been viewed as technologies of the self and perceived as part of a broader disciplinary regime (e.g., Foucault 1988; Rose 1999).

It is important to note that the medicalization thesis throughout its history has had either a gender-neutral or a female-gendered content (Riska 2003). At its inception, when Zola introduced the thesis, it had a gender-neutral meaning: it indicated a generic trend in modern medicine. The thesis soon came to have a gendered content when the women's health movement annexed it and used it as a lens through which to view the impact of high-tech medicine on women's bodies and health. The thesis enabled women to claim that women were the primary targets of the medicalization process.

Men's bodies were not described in terms of medicalization until well into the 1990s. At issue was the medical treatment of sexual dysfunction and hormone deficiency. The promotion of Viagra and drugs for men's alleged menopausal symptoms is an example of the trend (Marshall 2002). This kind of hormone theory of health had been a way of explaining women's mental-health problems in the nineteenth century (Theriot 1993, 24). During the past fifty years, hormone deficiency has been used to explain a wide range of chronic illnesses in women, ranging from osteoporosis to CHD.

A central theme of this book is that men's health has been medicalized in the past too, but in a different, less overt manner than women's health. Chapter 3 shows that in the 1950s and 1960s the traits of traditional masculinity were translated into a risk factor for men's developing CHD. At fifty years' distance, it could be argued that the construction of Type A as a medical risk factor came to conceal the crisis of masculinity, even for men. By medicalizing traditional masculinity, the underlying strains in the gender order and pressure for a behavioral and cultural change in men were translated into a medical issue. Medicine naturalized the sex-role strain for men and integrated the psychosomatic signs of the strain into its medical discourse. The crisis was transformed into the domain of the natural and handled by the domain of medicine, where it could be dealt with as unmarked by gender. In this way the category of Type A maintained men's gender as a natural and generic category. A naturalization of the pressure for a change in men's sex roles obscured the underlying gender, race, and class structure; and the embedded structural inequalities were thus not made transparent.

THE METHODOLOGICAL APPROACH

The analysis in this book uses a Foucault-inspired genealogical method (Armstrong 1990; Foucault 1975), the purpose of which is to trace the origin of three psychological categories: Type A personality, hardiness, and John Henryism. The task is to unpack the historical epistemology of these psychological categories (see Rose 1999, xiv). The analysis presented in the following chapters is social constructionist, a sociology-of-knowledge perspective represented by Danziger in his review of American psychology (1997). Danziger argues that the essence of psychological categories lies not so much in their reflection of "nature" but of historically constructed categories: "Historically, the big question about the category of 'personality' is how it ended up as a psychological category" (1997, 124). As he shows, the development of new psychological tests constructed the new psychological categories and enabled the mapping of the phenomenon. I show that the instruments—the scales developed—have both produced and confirmed the psychological categories—the various coronary-prone personalities—constructed in this way.

The data were collected through a Medline search from 1965 through 2002 to examine the pioneering articles and the subsequent use of the constructs. The constructs appear in texts that have produced and constructed the meaning of these psychological categories. These texts constitute part of the scientific discourse of psychology, but they are available in the form of scientific articles, a condition that makes them part of the public discourse (see Danziger 1997, 184). In 2002, there were 1,448 articles returned by a search for the phrase "Type A personality," 225 articles on hardiness as a protective factor for human health, and 22 articles on John Henryism. The analysis reported here is qualitative: it examines the scientific discovery of a certain type of personality assumed to explain the prevalence of CHD among American men. In focus are the methods and data sections of the scientific articles, which tell about the subjects of the research and the construction of the instruments. The sociological reading of these scientific texts constitutes a meta-analysis of the research design and the results reported in the articles.

CONCLUSION

The recent debates in the public health field on men's health disadvantages portray a reductionist picture of the reasons for men's health problems. This reductionism is characterized by psychologism and methodological individualism. Psychological reductionism implies that men's health is not interpreted as related to men's social behavior and social position as men, but as related to their "human nature," measured as a certain personality predisposition. Methodological individualism means that the psychological characteristics of individual men are used for explaining and predicting the rates of CHD in different groups of men, a rate that is a collective and social phenomenon.

The recent men's health discourse might eventually result in a broader awareness of the gendered aspects of men's health. The debate might signal a growing interest in a sociological understanding of men's gendered health. The purpose of this book is to provide the reader with analytical tools to see and understand men's health from such a gendered perspective. I aim to deconstruct the personality-focused etiological theories of CHD and to tease out the gendered man and the gendered character of this medical knowledge. This aim echoes the quest of British sociologist Alan Petersen for a more systematic analysis of how male bodies have been constructed through scientific and cultural practices and "how particular male bodies, namely the bodies of white, European, middle-class, heterosexual men, have been constructed as the standard for measuring and evaluating other bodies" (1998, 41). Translated to the American context, the task is to unravel the crucial role of science in making knowledge of the minds and bodies of white middle-class American men the standard and universal knowledge of heart disease. My argument is that the scientific discourses harbor notions about the moral character of middle-class men. Here we are reminded of the moral undertones in the risk-factor approach to chronic disease. Aronowitz has drawn attention to the concealed moral content of this kind of epidemiological thinking: "Increasingly, we believe or act as if any relationships between etiologic theories and the ideal moral order is merely coincidental fallout from truth-seeking medical research, rather than the congruence of similar belief systems" (1998, 178).

The personality theories on coronary disease do not only constitute a part of the epidemiological thinking about heart disease, but they also belong to broader social and philosophical theories. These theories grapple with a perennial issue in the history of thought in the modern era: the vision of a particular dominant character or personality felt to be essential for the maintenance of social order (Rieff 1959, 356, and 1966, 2; Susman 1984, 273; see also Devereux 1964; Connell 1987, 224). The typifications of personalities have therefore to be seen as a way to construct and confirm the moral and social order of men.

Here Michèle Lamont's terms *moral order* and *historical national repertoires* can serve as heuristic devices to understand the unique character of Type A in American public discourse (1992 and 2000, 136). In her qualitative study of upper-middle-class men in the United States and France in the early 1990s, Lamont found that there was an underlying consensus about some general values in each of these two countries, a consensus she called historical national repertoires. For example, the individualistic ethos was a basic theme in the United States, but there were also differences in the way that the men in each country presented themselves in the moral order: there was a typification system of what constituted the moral self. In fact, morality was a boundary-maintenance device used by men to define and constitute themselves in the class, gender, and racial order as men. Lamont shows that success, a work ethic, responsibility, self-actualization, and a "disciplined self" were key values in American men's cultural repertoire, in contrast to that of French men, for whom cultural values and cultural distinctions were more salient (1992, 130, and 2000, 26).

Chapter Three

The Rise of Type A Man
in Medical Discourse

At first sight there is something surprising in this strange unrest of so many happy men, restless in the midst of abundance. The spectacle itself, however, is as old as the world; the novelty is to see a whole people furnish an exemplification of it.

—Alexis de Tocqueville, *Democracy in America*

In biomedicine, disease is generally treated as a given natural category and the physician as a passive identifier of disease. Such a view conceptualizes the history of medicine as the achievements of great men, able to identify new diseases and confirm their etiology and, thereby, to improve the health and well-being of individuals and populations. Yet, the history of medicine can also be perceived as the tale of the rise and fall of medical discourses that have provided a lens through which the physician has constructed disease and its causes. As Cassell argues, the rise and fall of new concepts and viewpoints in medicine "are part of a larger change in the manner in which humanity views itself and its relationship to nature" (1986, 40).

For Foucault, biomedicine was a discourse that in the late eighteenth and the nineteenth century made visible new categories of disease theretofore disguised and hidden from the medical gaze (1975). Similarly, Armstrong argues that a new medical discourse—surveillance medicine—emerged in the mid-twentieth century, a discourse that problematized the so-called normal and healthy states of individuals (1995). This discourse identified new risk factors and lifestyles that put certain groups, and even whole populations, in an exceptional and perennial preillness at-risk state.

My focus is the construction of heart disease rates, which have been part of surveillance medicine and a way of watching over an increase in men's

27

deaths. By the 1960s, a new discourse emerged to explain men's high CHD rates: the personality-focused discourse. This discourse is reductionist because, like the stress discourse in later medical thinking (Young 1980, 142; Wainwright and Calnan 2002), it reduces all social structures and social processes to attributes of individuals. The psychological discourse was a gaze that revealed the "personality" of humans. It was here in this space of the deep self that the forces of the embodied self were hidden. This space of the self was conceptualized as a person's personality, and its identification enabled the localization of disease, especially heart disease. As Danziger notes about the moral overtones in the discovery of the concept of personality in American society, "Not only had 'personality' become a part of the individual that had to be watched anxiously for signs of disease, it had also become a universal possession capable of degrees of perfection defined in terms of a vocabulary of social effectiveness" (1997, 125).

The rise of the Type A construct in the mid-1950s became an important social category of surveillance medicine, a category that was used as a diagnostic instrument in predicting CHD. The Type A person has been characterized by a certain behavioral and personality pattern called "Type A behavior pattern" and "Type A personality." This was not a gender-neutral diagnostic category. As this chapter shows, Type A was constructed by medicalizing traditional masculinity. During the past decades, the death rate from CHD among men has fallen dramatically in most of the West. Yet, what happened to the Type A man? Having had the status of an independent medical risk factor in the late 1960s and most of the 1970s, Type A has all but disappeared as a social and diagnostic category in the vocabulary of medicine.

This chapter explores the rise of the Type A man. It examines the social construction of a certain type of masculinity introduced as a significant risk factor for developing CHD, in the medical literature in the late 1950s.

The method of the analysis reported here is genealogical (Armstrong 1990): the aim is to find the origin and development of the concept of the Type A man in modern medical discourse. The mapping was done by collecting the material via the Medline computer database. Both a quantitative and qualitative analysis was conducted of the scientific references to the topic listed in Medline (i.e., U.S. National Library of Medicine 2003). The qualitative analysis focused on the early scientific articles introducing this term and on later articles and books specifying the characteristics of the behavior displayed by Type A men. The count yielded 1,448 entries on "Type A personality" from 1965 through 2002 (1,387 if analyzed as a MeSH-term). No entries on "Type A" or "Type A behavioral pattern" were found. The absence of entries on the latter two concepts relates to the lack of use of these terms as key phrases in Medline, a finding that is in itself interesting. Medline, a medical literature search system, traces literature back to 1966, and the key phrase "Type A personality" (which overlaps with coronary-prone personality) was introduced into the search system in 1985 (U.S. National Library of Medicine 1998, 1214). Entries before 1985 cannot be considered to provide as complete coverage as the references after 1985.

THE SELF-MADE MAN BECOMES TYPE A MAN

In the words of Foucault, "the space of configuration" of a disease has to be laid down before the space of localization of the illness can be seen and explained (1975, 3). CHD, at least its location, was seen by the medical gaze long before a search for its prevention began. At the hands of the pioneers of biomedicine, behavioral typing became a way of identifying the person who was to succumb to CHD. As early as 1910, Sir William Osler pondered why angina pectoris was more common in the upper classes: "It is as though only a special strain of tissue reacted anginally, so to speak, a type evolved amid special surroundings or which existed in certain families" (1910, 839). He then offered a prescientific version of a Type A behavior:

> It is not the delicate neurotic person who is prone to angina, but the robust, the vigorous in mind and body, and the keen and ambitious man, the indicator of whose engines is always at "full speed ahead." There is, indeed, a frame and facies at once suggestive of angina—the well "set" man of from 45 to 55 years of age, with military bearing, iron-grey hair, and florid complexion. (Osler 1910, 839)

A number of habits and behaviors, encapsulating the lifestyles of a consumerist society, was later added to the list constructed by epidemiologists, who began to explore the risk factors related to the prevalence of CHD among men. Coronary-prone men were not randomly distributed. In post–World War II Western society, they occupied the more affluent social positions. These men's typical lifestyle—in particular, smoking and overeating—came first in the listing of medical risk factors.

After World War II, the first to spot the physical and psychological weakness of Western men were those concerned with the obesity of American men. While the picture of fat capitalists, resembling ambulatory moneybags, had been derided early in the century, the plight of the nation's obese men was taken to heart in the 1950s. As Berrett shows, the dieting man was a cultural concept hard to promote since the image of dieting was connected with feminine values (1997). Hence, the discourse on the dieting American man touted the restoration of traditional masculine values of self-control and a rebuttal of the values of an other-directed consumerist society represented by its alluring fatty and sugar-filled food.

While large surveys on male populations tended to show that smoking and obesity were the major medical risk factors for developing CHD, there were also studies that failed to confirm the association. By the early 1960s, the medical gaze turned to men's interiors—their selves and their masculinity—and a new risk factor was discovered. For long, the inner self of men had been the essentialist core of masculinity. The picture of normative masculinity was a man who was in control, both of his inner self and of his environment. The "silent masculine mystique" has implied a valorization of men's inner life (Berrett 1997, 819; Nonn 1995); yet, it could only exist as a male asset as long as it was compared to the opposite gender and the assumed emotional character of women.

In the early 1950s, a classic in the sociological literature, C. Wright Mills's *White Collar: The American Middle Classes* (1951), alerted the scientific community to the unique social position and cultural disposition of the new postwar American middle class. As Mills suggested, white-collared people "carry, in a most revealing way, many of those psychological themes that characterize our epoch" (1951, iv). This social class was to be the target of sociological research for reasons Mills suggests:

> We need to characterize American society of the mid-twentieth century in more psychological terms, for now the problems that concern us most border on the psychiatric. It is one great task of social studies today to describe the larger economic and political situation in terms of its meaning for the inner life and the external career of the individual, and in doing this to take into account how the individual often becomes falsely conscious and blinded. In the welter of the individual's daily experience the framework of modern society must be sought; within that framework the psychology of the little man must be formulated. (1951, xx)

Mainstream sociologists mapped the behavior of the very same middle-class men in the mid-1950s and proclaimed the traditional male sex-role behavior functional for the family and society (Parsons and Bales 1955). The functionalist view of the family presented a reciprocal pattern of male and female sex roles (i.e., men taking on the instrumental tasks, and women the expressive tasks). Nevertheless, the demands on the male role were such that they could put a man in a stressful position. In the early 1940s, Parsons, perhaps still having the Great Depression and its threats fresh in mind, observed:

> It is of fundamental significance to the sex role structure of the adult age levels that the normal man has a "job" which is fundamental to his social status in general. It is perhaps not too much to say that only in very exceptional cases can an adult man be genuinely self-respecting and enjoy a respected status in the eyes of others if he does not "earn a living" in an approved occupation. (1942, 608)

When the traditional male sex-role characteristics were seen through the lens of medicine, they were, however, declared a health hazard. The traditional masculinity of the American middle-class man was assigned a medical term, *Type A behavior pattern*. It was towards these "new little Machiavellians" (Mills 1951, xvii) that the medical community turned its medical gaze and thereafter found Type A man.

THE MEDICALIZATION OF TRADITIONAL MASCULINITY

In the mid-1950s, two American cardiologists, Meyer Friedman and Ray Rosenman, who worked at the Harold Brunn Institute of Mount Zion Hospital and Medical Center in San Francisco, became interested in the stress-related patterns of behavior of their cardiac patients. In their own words, it all began in 1954, when "the idea was born that a person's feelings and thoughts have an influence on the development of coronary heart disease" (Friedman and Ulmer 1984, 4). This idea had its origin in a very concrete piece of evidence in the chairs in the reception room of the two cardiologists: the front edges of the upholstery of the chair seats were worn out (Friedman and Rosenman 1974, 55). This upholstery sign, the cardiologists recall in retrospect, indicated the unique behavioral pattern of their clients. A later survey of male managers' thoughts about what kind of habits precipitated a heart attack led the researchers down a new trail in medical thinking. The new trail resulted in the unfolding of a specific behavioral pattern that was assumed to be an indicator of the emotions of their male clients. In 1956 and 1957 the group reported some preliminary studies on "emotional stress" and "excessive competitive drive" (e.g., Friedman et al., 1958), and a more systematic study of the phenomenon was initiated.

Nevertheless, a grant proposal on the topic was turned down twice in the review conducted by the National Institutes of Health (NIH), but the research group was eventually encouraged to change the terminology related to the expected key independent variable on emotions. As Friedman recalls, the NIH representative, Dr. C. J. Van Slyke, suggested in 1958 that "the specific emotion-action complex which we had observed in coronary patients be called Type A behavior pattern" because, Van Slyke indicated, "such a description I don't believe will annoy the psychiatrists reviewing your grant applications" (1977, 593–594). The third time it was submitted, now with the new terminology, the grant was approved. Obviously, Van Slyke's suggestion was an apt one since the more descriptive and neutral term, derived from the three study groups to be examined, A, B, and C, was stripped of any association with psychological or psychiatric theory. Friedman and Rosenman were, foremost, clinicians whose medical gaze derived from their own office experience with patients, a method they called "behavioral typing." Although their approach gave the impression at first glance of being as neutral as classifying butterflies according to color, at issue was not a random selection of individuals: employed, white, middle-class, middle-aged men were the target of their studies.

At issue were two simultaneous health problems in the United States in the 1950s: the high prevalence of stress and of CHD among middle-class white-collar men. The medical community spotted these syndromes as the "executive disease," as CHD was sometimes called then, and attributed them to the special lifestyle of these men. The stress syndrome was also dubbed "hurry sickness" in some medical circles (e.g., Friedman and Rosenman 1974, 70) to indicate the fast pace and drive of men holding the executive positions in mid-twentieth-century America. Soon a proper medical diagnosis was found: these were Type A men. Friedman and Rosenman, in their seminal article in *The Journal of the American Medical Association* (*JAMA*) in 1959, defined the type:

> A person was adjudged as exhibiting completely developed behavior pattern A if he exhibited various signs we believed indicative of its presence, including excessively rapid body movements, tense facial and body musculature, explosive conversational intonations, hand or teeth clenching, excessive unconscious gesturing, and a general air of impatience, and if he admitted his sustained drive, competitiveness, and necessity to accelerate many activities and was aware of a chronic sense of urgency in daily living. (1959, 1287)

This was the first time that the term *Type A behavior* was used in a scientific article. This "overt behavior pattern," designated A, consisted of six characteristics:

> 1) an intense, sustained drive to achieve self-selected but usually poorly defined goals, 2) profound inclination and eagerness to compete, 3) persistent desire for recognition and advancement, 4) continuous involvement in multiple and diverse functions constantly subject to time restrictions (deadlines), 5) habitual propensity to accelerate the rate of execution of many physical and mental functions, and 6) extraordinary mental and physical alertness. (Friedman and Rosenman 1959, 1286)

A series of empirical studies was undertaken to test the relationship between these behaviors, certain emotions, and the propensity to develop CHD.

The three study groups were called group A (overt behavior pattern A), group B (overt behavior pattern B), and group C (overt behavior pattern C). Selected for group A were eighty-three men from "engineering, paper manufacturing, and aluminum corporations, newspaper organizations, advertising agencies, grocery chains, television stations, and other independent businesses"—largely, various types of executives (Friedman and Rosenman 1959, 1287). These men had been recruited by means of a method that, sociologically speaking, could be called "reputational technique." The researchers approached some people working in the areas of choice, who then selected colleagues who fitted the description of behavior pattern A. Similarly, selected for group B were eighty-three men from an employees' union of a municipal government, a union of professional embalmers, and twelve accounting firms. Group C comprised forty-six unemployed blind men who were assumed to have "little ambition, drive, or desire to compete" because of their blindness, but still to live in "a chronic state of insecurity and anxiety" due to their financial and physical insecurity (Friedman and Rosenman 1959, 1287). The researchers concluded:

> Men of group A exhibited a behavior pattern primarily characterized by intense ambition, competitive "drive," constant preoccupation with occupational "deadlines," and a sense of time urgency and the men of group B, a converse behavior pattern. Men of group C exhibited a behavior pattern essentially similar to that exhibited by men of group B, but with the added elements of a chronic anxiety state. (Friedman and Rosenman 1959, 1295)

The authors observed that clinical artery disease was seven times more frequent and *arcus senilis* over three times more frequent in the men of group A than in those of group B or group C. The results, the authors concluded, "strongly suggest that the behavior pattern exhibited by the men of group A was of itself largely responsible" for the incidence of disease (Friedman and Rosenman 1959, 1295).

A year later, Friedman and Rosenman again published an article in the *Journal of the American Medical Association* further exploring the assumption that detection and recognition of "behavior pattern A in individual or groups of persons might be expected to have considerable prognostic as well as diagnostic value" (1960, 1320). For this purpose, they had designed a "psychophysiological test" composed of the taped recordings of two monologues, one spoken by a man and another by a woman. The researchers described their instrument as follows:

> The male monologue, *serving as a control* and requiring 942 seconds for its complete audition, consisted of a discussion of the various factors generally considered essential for vocational success. It was delivered evenly, relatively rapidly, and forcefully by a strong masculine voice.
>   This second monologue, *designed as the experimental challenge* monologue, deliberately and repetitively dealt with a trivial, nonsensical subject. It was delivered extraordinarily slowly and very hesitantly by a soft but pleasant feminine voice. The repetitive nature of the latter discussion quickly permitted the listener

to foretell the end of each sentence a few seconds before it was actually spoken. (Friedman and Rosenman 1960, 1321–1322; italics added)

Three groups characterized by pattern A, B, and C behavior were subject to a Reid-type polygraph that recorded the subjects' respiratory and body movements and "any possible hand-clenching occurring" (Friedman and Rosenman 1960, 1321). The readings of the polygraph indicated that thirteen of the twenty patients with CHD had high scores and that "such reactions, moreover, appeared far more frequently during the portions of the slow female monologue" (Friedman and Rosenman 1960, 1322). A rationale for why their major indicators—the two monologues—had a built-in gender bias was not offered in the methods section or in the reporting of the results. The reader of the article is confronted with a given fact that was in all likelihood so taken for granted by the researchers that it needed no further explication in the contemporary gender environment.

Friedman and Rosenman embarked the same year on a more ambitious project with a larger population basis and a follow-up design. This was the Western Collaborative Group Study that initially included 3,524 healthy, white middle- and upper-level male executives employed in 10 California companies, 39 to 59 years old, who were examined from June 1960 to December 1961 and then for 8.5 years. At the beginning of the study, the men at risk ($n = 3,154$) were classified as either the tense Type A ($n = 1,589$) or as the more relaxed Type B ($n = 1,565$).

In the report of the findings of the first part of the study after four and a half years, the researchers seem to have a greater confidence in their theory, and they use the term *Type A men*. They conclude, for example, that "in each such comparison *Type A men* suffered higher CHD rates than did men with the converse Type B behavior pattern" (italics added; Rosenman et al., 1970, 189). A more general description of the results was reported in *Hospital Practice* in 1971, which also gave a clear definition of what was now called Type A man:

As his responses indicate, the type A person is invariably punctual and greatly annoyed if kept waiting; he rarely finds time to indulge in hobbies, and when he does, he makes them as competitive as his vocation. He dislikes helping at home in routine jobs because he feels that his time can be spent more profitably. He walks rapidly, eats rapidly, and rarely remains long at the dinner table. He often tries to do several things at once and carries a second line of thought if he can possibly manage it. (Rosenman and Friedman 1971, 90)

Friedman and Rosenman called this a behavior pattern, because "it is an overt and observable pattern that reflects an individual's characteristic responses" that the individual may not be aware of (Rosenman 1978, 60).

The predictive power of the Type A behavioral pattern came from the final results of the Western Collaborative Group Study. After eight and a half years, the follow-up of a sample of seemingly healthy middle-aged men found that twice as many Type A as Type B men developed heart disease (Rosenman et al., 1975). The innovative feature of the Type A model was that the two cardiology clinicians had developed a method of diagnosing Type A behavior among healthy men, and they had demonstrated that Type A behavioral pattern could be used to predict CHD. The predictive instrument was the so-called Structured Interview, an interview schedule of twenty-seven questions that elicited those behaviors that the clinicians had seen as indicative of the emotions harbored by a coronary-prone person. This interview method they perceived as more objective than any self-reports through a questionnaire because the assessment of the behavior pattern "is far better based on the observations of a trained observer rather than upon the opinion of the subject" (Rosenman 1978, 60; see interview schedule, 68–69).

On the basis of the responses to the Structured Interview, a person would be classified as a fully developed Type A (A-1), incompletely developed Type A (A-2), midway between A and B (X), or definitely non-A (B). In his review of the interview method and how to spot the profile of behavior pattern Type A, Rosenman provides the following characterization of "the extreme Type A person," or Type A-1:

> The Type A-1 individual walks briskly. His face looks extraordinarily alert; that is, his eyes are very much alive, more quickly seeking to take in the situation at a glance. He may employ a tense, teeth-clenching, and jaw-grinding posture. His smile has a lateral extension rather than an oval, and his laughter is rarely a "belly-laugh." He tends to look you straight and quite unflinchingly in the eye. He frequently sits poised on the edge of a chair. He may stretch out his feet, cross them, or just keep them bent under his chair. (1978, 61)

When he interacts, a Type A person will gesticulate in a special way:

> Rarely do his hands hang limply, with fingers widely spaced. He is apt, whenever he is *enthused* about a subject, to gesture, and particularly, to clench his fist. He will rarely clench his fist as you talk, only when he talks, and then particularly when enthused and excited or when angry and upset. He is apt to give you the impression that he is impatient, and even more, he may make you feel slightly uneasy in your own slowness when you are near him. (Rosenman 1978, 61)

But his way of talking is also revealing that he is a Type A:

> His speech is not necessarily fast, but often may carry explosive intonations and it accelerates in longer sentences. He tends to put punch in key words of a sentence.

He never whines, rarely talks in a whisper and rarely pauses in the middle of sentences. If he begins to talk about a subject that interests him, and if he is interrupted, usually he will bring the conversation back to the subject that interested him or where he was talking when he was interrupted. (Rosenman 1978, 61)

And furthermore in his relations to his family, he is characterized by impatience:

He hates to lose any sort of contest, even with his own children. "When I play a game, I play to win," and then he might add, "Isn't that what a game is for?" He does not like to do routine things around the house, like cleaning dishes, mopping floors, cleaning, etc. He usually does not like to garden. In short, anything that does not appear to be a worthwhile achievement leaves him cold. (Rosenman 1978, 62)

After a detailed listing of a number of masculine attributes, the conclusion is that "after many years of a competitive, driving, unending quest for constantly receding goals, the Type A-1 subject exhibits mannerisms and various motor actions that very often allow him to be identified" (Rosenman 1978, 62). These behavioral responses are believed to be determined "by the interplay of the individual's own personality facade with the demands, stresses, and distresses of his own environmental milieu, both vocational and avocational" (Rosenman 1978, 60).

In a popularized version of their research findings, a book entitled *Type A Behavior and Your Heart*, Friedman and Rosenman described in detail the characteristics of the "fully developed, hard-core Type A," a man "aggressively involved in a chronic, incessant struggle to achieve more and more in less and less time" (Friedman and Rosenman 1974, 67). This "drive to self-destruction" Friedman and Rosenman saw as a personality characteristic rather than as tied to a specific moment in American economic development when the small entrepreneur was struggling to survive in a tidal wave of emerging corporate capitalism (1974, 40). They described this individualistic attribute and seemingly irrational work ethic in the following terms:

Type A behavior is above all a continuous struggle, an unremitting attempt to accomplish or achieve more and more things or participate in more and more events in less and less time, frequently in the face of opposition—real or imagined— from other persons. The Type A personality is dominated by covert insecurity of status or hyper-aggressiveness, or both. (1974, 31)

The new medical gaze yielded the Type A behavioral pattern, but the researchers humbly referred to the new knowledge as deriving from their clinical expertise rather than annexing psychology to their new discourse:

We are not psychologists. What follows is an honest description of symptoms and signs as we have observed them. . . . It is possible that our *psychological* analysis may be criticized as superficial, perhaps rightly so. But this by no means invalidates its medical significance. The Type A man is prone to heart disease; these characteristic behavioral habits identify the Type A man. (Friedman and Rosenman 1974, 69)

The listed characteristic behavioral habits were gendered. According to Friedman and Rosenman, women were still sheltered from the competitive economic environment of the public domain, an environment that fostered Type A man: "There are comparatively few Type A American white females as completely immersed as males in the contemporary economic and professional milieu that nourishes the development of Type A Behavior Pattern" (1974, 62).

But as other researchers later noted in a study of female secretaries conducted to spot Type A behavior among women, "With regard to Type A behavior, hard-driving, competitive, and hostile behaviors are unlikely to lead to material rewards in secretaries. Similarly, the job is noticeably lacking in control and challenge" (Schmied and Lawler 1986, 1222).

But the cardiologist pair—Friedman and Rosenman—had also stumbled on another pertinent health issue: the inequality of health. While the pattern of heart disease took its toll differently from the one now associated with the debate about health inequality, the same undercurrent of morality was still involved. Why would hard-working male breadwinners devoted to the values of American work ethic be punished by nature?

Three genuinely sociological notions were transparent in the idea of the overt behavior pattern A. First, this concept recognized emotions to be what Williams called the "missing link" between structure and agency, mind and body, biology and society (1998, 126). The term implied a recognition that certain men could not be understood as merely biological or disembodied beings, but rather had to be conceptualized by their position in the social structure and as existentially embodied and gendered people.

Second, the behavioral display of anger, hostility, and aggression by Type A men was medically diagnosed as pathological, rather than as constituting part of the normal registry of violence associated with traditional masculinity. The Type A thesis contained an indirect critique of men's aggressive behavior and challenged the normalization of violence embedded in the dominant form of masculinity.

Third, the new medical gaze on modern middle-class men implied what Ehrenreich has called "a rewriting of the masculine script" (1983, 68). Behaviors that had been perceived as physical and moral virtues in middle-class men—working hard, striving for achievement, taking responsibility, competing—were suddenly recast as emotions that were presented as a health hazard for the very same men. The high rate of CHD among middle-class men now constituted "the cost of masculinity" (Messner 1997, 6): a realization that conformity to a narrow definition of masculinity could be lethal for men.

The rewriting of the masculine script was based on a paradox: middle-class men were too aggressive and hard working and, therefore, were psychologically vulnerable. The conformity of white American middle-class breadwinners to the work ethic landed them with a medical label for their trouble: they were Type A men.

WHO ARE THE TYPE B AND TYPE C MEN?

The Characteristics of Type B Men

In the original research by Friedman and Rosenman, the Type B construct remained a residual category. Type B was a non-A type (see p. 35). The earliest description of the traits characterizing Type B is found in the original inventors' portrayal of "pattern B" that was "characterized by relative absence of drive, ambition, sense of urgency, desire to compete, or involvement in deadlines" (Friedman and Rosenman 1959, 1286). A man was classified as a "completely developed behavior pattern B" if he "sat relaxedly, moved slowly and calmly, exhibited no muscular tension, spoke slowly, rarely indulged in tense gestures, exhibited no impatience, and denied even moderate drive or ambition, shunned competition, avoided involvement in deadlines, and felt no sense of urgency" (Friedman and Rosenman 1959, 1287).

In a later guide to spotting Type A and B men in clinical practice, Rosenman provided detailed behavioral characterizations of the two types (1978). The guide alerted the clinician about how to use the Structured Interview method to assess a variety of behavioral patterns among men. Rosenman portrays Type B man as follows:

> A true "B" is one who from earliest days never cared to compete excessively or to run a race with time. Of course, he might have been a good student and even a superb thinker. He might work long hours and be very conscientious but usually he does not feel the need to compress events in time enough "each day." . . . He cuts a smaller piece of the pie of life. He is not apt to relinquish vacations or take up night school studies for his advancement. He is often very satisfied with his status, both economic and social. He never makes one think of the sharply discharged arrow. He ambles along; he does not run. His whole demeanor suggests relaxation, unhurriedness, and contentment. (1978, 64)

In social interaction the Type B man's facial expressions will reveal his inner calm and emotional stability. Rosenman describes him as follows: "The face of the Type B person is relaxed in expression, lacks muscle rigidity and with relaxed lips. His smile is apt to be broader and his mouth forms roundedness when he laughs. He may have an intelligent face; no hostility is seen" (1978, 64).

Rosenman further describes the behavioral pattern of Type B:

> He usually tends to relax by sitting back in a chair. You have the idea he is sitting in the chair to remain there and does not seem to regard it as a launching pad or pierced with small nails. His hands usually hang loosely, fingers outstretched; he never clenches his fist. He will shake your hand relatively gently, although in nervousness, he might shake it frequently and rapidly. (1978, 64)

Type B is relaxed towards his work and activities outside work, or as Rosenman suggests, "He has no guilt feelings about nonachievement-oriented activities. . . . He is apt to do more routine things around the house, apt to garden more, to have hobbies that carry no great goal or purpose" (1978, 65). At work Type B is characterized by a rational work style and an ability to delegate tasks: "His work record will not be particularly distinguished if he is a laborer, but if he is high echelon, his very ability to sit back and think and to delegate may have moved him along high in corporate status. Many top executives, for example, are Type B" (Rosenman 1978, 65).

The influence of the environment can turn some Type B people into Type A-2, which is the "less overt, less exaggerated A type behavior pattern." Rosenman pondered the possibilities: "You can visualize that a relaxed, basically Type B personality becomes Type A if the individual works on an assembly line, is paid on the basis of 'piece work,' or drives a taxi cab in modern urban environments" (1978, 63).

Aside from these individual attributes, there is an indirect economic definition of Type B men in the selected samples in the pioneering studies: Type B men were salaried and worked for large organizations (see Friedman and Rosenman 1959, 1287). The characteristics are shared between the samples collected for testing Type B and for testing the later construct of hardiness: both samples included salaried and white-collar male workers. This social position gave Type B men and the hardy executive some economic protection against the blind forces of entrepreneurial capitalism that was the terrain to conquer and survive in for the self-made man of the Type A stripe.

Type B was used in the later Framingham Heart Study, a study reviewed in the end of this chapter. In this study Type A behavior was measured by the Framingham Type A Behavior Scale (see chapter 7). For the purpose of that study, Type As were defined as people scoring in the upper 50 percent of the scale and Type Bs were those scoring in the lower 50 percent (Haynes et al., 1978b, 387; Eaker et al., 1983, 25).

In the 1990s, there emerged a new interest in the neglected Type B man. For example, Kaplan urged researchers to take a closer look at "the neglected Type B construct—a hypothesized style of health-promoting personal and striving skills" (1992, 4), although others have deplored the lack of psychological theory underlying the Type B concept (Friedman 1990, 285).

The Characteristics of Type C Men

Scant information about Type C men was given in the original study conducted by Friedman and Rosenman. In the pioneering article in 1959, Friedman and Rosenman defined the third "pattern C" as "characterized by its similarity to pattern B but also including a chronic state of anxiety or insecurity" (p. 1286). The original operationalization of pattern C gave no specific behavioral characteristics of Type C men for what the researchers considered a simple reason: "a ubiquitous general air of resignation, worry, and hopelessness" in these men (Friedman and Rosenman 1959, 1287). Why the latter psychosocial conditions were not considered stressors and a health hazard was not explained.

In the empirical testing of their hypothesis about behavioral pattern A, selected for group C were forty-six blind men assumed to have "little ambition, drive, or desire to compete" because of their blindness and unemployment. Furthermore, they were assumed to live in "a chronic state of insecurity and anxiety" due to their financial and physical insecurity (Friedman and Rosenman 1959, 1287). The original definition of Type C men fits the contemporary stereotypical culture-of-poverty ideal type constructed in social science literature, which portrayed poor inner-city men as having no ambition or drive and living in a subculture of poverty characterized by resignation and hopelessness (see Rose 1972, 41–50).

No reference to Type C is made in Friedman and Rosenman's later work. Type C is constructed as a marginalized man in the American gender and economic hierarchy, and at that time it seems he was of little interest to medical science.

Almost twenty-five years later Type C was rehabilitated and used in research on cancer. Type C has been defined as a "cancer-prone personality." This construct is used for portraying a gloomy personality: "The Type C individual may be seen as chronically hopeless and helpless" (Temoshok 1987, 558). Furthermore, Type C has been presented as a personality that represents a cooperative, unassertive, nonverbal, and low emotionality style—the opposite of the active and impatient Type A pattern (e.g. Temoshok et al., 1985, 141–142). A vivid description of Type C suggests the following traits: "The Type C individual is considered nice, friendly and helpful to others, and rarely gets into arguments or fights; this is the person one likes to have as a neighbour, or to organize the local charity drive" (Temoshok 1987, 558). Nevertheless, the problem of Type C is that this person does not express his or her feelings, but has what is defined as an inhibited style. As Temoshok suggests, "The Type C individual does not even try to express needs and feelings; these are hidden under a mask of normalcy and self-sufficiency" (1987, 560).

A later review on personality and health has specified the characteristics of Type C vis-à-vis Type A in the following way: "Central to the proposed 'Type C' construct is the nonexpression and/or nonexperience of negative emotion, particularly anger. Just as the Type A individual is angry, hostile, and explosive, the Type C person does not report anger and presents a pleasant, cheerful, or impassive face to the world" (Contrada et al., 1990, 658).

As the description of the Type A man in the previous section of this chapter and the foregoing portrayals of Type B and C show, the maleness of these categories is taken for granted in the original definition of these constructs. It is in this sense that gender is an invisible category in the construction of Type A, B, and C as diagnostic categories. The whiteness of these categories of masculinities is also taken for granted in two respects. First, the original studies did not include African American men in the samples. Second, the description and analysis of Type A men did not locate these men in their privileged position in the existing racial and ethnic hierarchies of superordination and subordination. Type A men were unmarked by gender and race. Their position in the racialized social order, like their position in the gender order, was taken for granted in the America of the 1950s, where the binary notion and value hierarchy of race and gender were still unchallenged. Later, research on personality factors that were viewed as medical risk factors for cardiovascular disease among African American men had to invent a new term: John Henryism (see chapter 6).

CHANGES IN THE GENDER ORDER: THE MEDICAL RISK FACTOR OF A WORKING SPOUSE FOR TYPE A AND B MEN

There is a genre of American health and medical research on Type A and CHD that has argued that women's liberation and the entry of women into the workforce have introduced a new and serious medical risk to men's health: the working spouse. In current public rhetoric this notion underlies the discourse on the crisis of masculinity (Kimmel and Kaufman 1995; Connell 2000; Whitehead 2002). It is assumed that changes in the economy and concomitant changes in the gender order pose a challenge for men to fulfill their function as men. It is assumed that this circumstance will take its toll in psychological and physical health costs for men.

This theme emerged early in the CHD and stress literature. The Framing-ham Heart Study conducted in the mid-1960s issued two major reports on the extensive study of the impact of the wife's status as housewife or as working wife on the husband's health. The studies set out to explore a number of questions related to this issue: for example, "Are certain behaviors among women associated with the development of heart disease in their husbands?" and "Are the incidence rates of heart disease among Type A men, as compared to Type B, modified by the social status and/or behaviors of their wives?" (Haynes et al., 1983, 2).

A set of 269 spouse pairs were used from the Framingham Heart Study cohort studied in 1965 and 1967 and followed over a 10-year period for the development of heart disease. The results showed that the mere fact that a man was married to a woman with a higher education constituted a considerable health risk, or as the reporting of the findings stated, "In general, men were at higher risk of developing coronary heart disease if married to a more educated woman, regardless of their own level of education" (Haynes et al., 1983, 10). For example, men with a grammar school education were 4.4 times more likely to develop heart disease if married to women with more education. In addition, the medical risk increased if the wife had some higher-level education (i.e., thirteen or more years of education). The health hazard of an educated wife was operationalized in rather biased terms: the presence of a highly educated spouse; or, as the findings stated, "men married to working women with 13 or more years of education . . . were 7.6 times more likely to develop heart disease than men married to women with a grammar school education" (Haynes et al., 1983, 12). The report concludes, "Men married to working women with an education beyond the high school level and to women employed in white-collar professions are at significantly higher risk of developing heart disease than men married to women of lower status" (Haynes et al., 1983, 17).

The Framingham Heart Study also explored how Type A and B men's health was influenced by the educational and labor-market status of their wives. The study's inquiry phrased the question as follows: "Is the risk of developing coronary heart disease among Type A men, as compared to B men, modified by the behavior or social status of their wives?" (Eaker et al., 1983, 24). As the researchers suggested, a "low stress situation" was one characterized by marriage to a housewife or a less-educated woman (Eaker et al., 1983, 39). In particular the researchers set out to explore "whether characteristics of wives could be viewed as *environmental stressors* and if they contributed to or modified the rates of coronary disease among Type A and Type B men" (emphasis added; Eaker et al., 1983, 29).

The study showed that Type A men were indeed at significantly higher risk of developing heart disease if married to women with thirteen or more years of education. Type A men were 2.5 times more likely to develop CHD than were Type B men with similarly educated wives. Furthermore, a working wife posed a far greater risk for Type A man than for Type B man: "Type A men had essentially the same rate of coronary disease as Type B men if married to housewives. . . . However, Type A men had 3.5 times the rate of heart disease as Type B men if they were married to working women" (Eaker et al., 1983, 31).

It is worth noting, however, that the early findings from the Framingham Heart Study had shown that "Type A working women and Type A housewives had an increased incidence of CHD as compared to their Type B counterparts" (Haynes et al., 1980, 56). But what impact would that have on their husbands' health? What if the wife was as hard working as her husband and showed characteristics measured as Type A among men? In this case the researchers postulated that "having a Type A wife would place a Type A husband at increased risk of developing heart disease because of the potential risk that such a marital arrangement might have on a husband's sense of control and self-esteem" (Eaker et al., 1983, 33). The "environmental stressor" of this lethal combination seemed evident to the researchers. Nevertheless, the researchers were slightly perplexed to note that Type A men were more at risk if they were married to Type B women than to Type A women. This unexpected result is given the following interpretation in the scientific reporting of the findings: "It might be psychologically and physiologically taxing for a husband who is hard-driving, competitive, and ambitious to live with a woman who is the opposite" (Eaker et al., 1983, 40).

The foregoing findings might be seen at twenty years' distance as mere expressions of an archaic scientific enterprise. Nevertheless, the same arguments have been presented in recent stress literature. A decade later, the "health costs" of wives' employment on husbands' psychological well-being continue to be in the focus of American stress research. For example, an article in *Journal of Health and Social Behavior* in 1992 reports the findings of an American study that confirmed that "insofar as it decreases husbands' relative income and increases their share of domestic labor, women's employment is negative for husbands' mental health" (Rosenfield 1992, 213).

CONCLUSION

The approach of the analysis reported in this chapter is Foucauldian (1975): it explores the genesis of a disease—CHD—and how its cause was defined and understood through the concept of Type A man. Type A man became a medical discourse that unveiled the scientific cause of CHD, a truth that had not been seen before, but was constructed after World War II into the major cause of CHD. The emotional factors involved were seen by two pioneers in the field, the cardiologists Meyer Friedman and Ray Rosenman, as inscribed in the surface of the body: a certain behavior pattern, named pattern A, was the sign of those emotions. But both the behaviors and the related emotional components were not neutral to class, race, or gender. At issue was a certain type of white middle-class masculinity that had up to then served as the normative guideline for male behavior: the behavior of the hard-working, achievement-oriented, and responsible male breadwinner. A glance at the display of this traditional form of masculinity by means of "behavioral typing" yielded the Type A man, dangerous to his own health. From a sociological point of view, the new medical discourse provided a fresh understanding of the gendered man as compared to the universal man that prevailed in the biological and pathological discourse reigning in biomedicine.

The rise of Type A man as a medical construct happened at a time that signaled two changes in society. One was a change in etiological thinking about CHD. The introduction of emotional factors as medical risk factors meant an infusion of new elements into the etiological thinking of the biomedical discourse of post-Flexnerian American medicine. Type A man was a new model of disease etiology that enabled physicians to recognize the emotional aspects of the key killer of men—CHD.

The second change was economic. The Depression and World War II changed the scene for the previously dominant economic actors: white professional men. In his examination of this social class of postwar men, C. Wright Mills noted, "Part of the new entrepreneur's frenzy perhaps is due to apprehension that his function may disappear" (1951, 99). For Mills, a decline of the power and status of the old middle class had taken place. The free entrepreneurs had lost their control over work and been succeeded by employees. As Mills saw it, this change "paralleled the decline of the independent individual and the rise of the little man in the American mind" (1951, xii).

In his portrayal of the psychological anxiety of the white-collar men of this period, Mills offers a clear diagnosis of the anxieties of Type A man:

> The new Little Man seems to have no firm roots, no sure loyalties to sustain his life and give it a center. He is not aware of having any history, his past being as brief as it is unheroic; he has lived through no golden age he can recall in time of trouble. Perhaps because he does not know where he is going, he is in a frantic hurry; perhaps because he does not know what frightens him, he is paralyzed with fear. (1951, xvi)

In this regard, the high level of aggression, hostility, and anger—called by a later group of health researchers the "AHA! syndrome" (Johnson and Spielberger 1992, 3)—was a general sign of the anxiety and mental distress of American middle-class men of the 1950s. The discourse on anxiety and stress in later psychological research might have been indicators of a loss of the control and power that this group of new Little Men felt in the prevailing race, class, and gendered hierarchies. The psychology of this Little Man became the focus of a new phase in the research on Type A man. As the next chapter shows, the coronary-prone Type A personality became the construct of a new psychological discourse on Type A man.

Chapter Four

The Fall of Type A Man: The Psychologization of the Concept

TYPE A MAN GETS A PERSONALITY

Back in 1957 it had been obvious to the psychiatrists reviewing the research proposal of the two pioneering cardiologists that the research project lacked a theory related to the independent variable on emotions. For Meyer Friedman and Ray Rosenman, observable behaviors served as indicators of the emotions of Type A man. In their view, a recorded relation between certain behaviors and the occurrence of CHD was enough to establish the "coronary-prone person."

The original measurement of Type A behavior was done by means of an instrument called the Structured Interview developed by Friedman and Rosenman (see Rosenman 1978). The Structured Interview consisted of twenty-seven questions about daily activities. The basic idea was that the interviewer should be authoritative and confront the subject by questioning or interrupting a response in order to deliberately challenge the subject and make him irritated and upset. The content of the subject's response was of less interest than how the subject expressed the responses and what kind of behaviors were displayed in the interaction. The Structured Interview instrument has been described as "a measure of behavioral reactivity to standardized psychosocial stress tasks" (Roskies 1987, 9). In other words, the interviewer records not only the attitudinal responses, but pays special attention to the behavioral responses—speech and motor behavior—to the questions (Matthews and Haynes 1986, 924–925; Edwards 1991, 152; Contrada et al., 1990, 647). This way of thinking was plagued by a certain essentialism, which could be phrased as, It is the nature of Type A people to produce Type A behavior (Young 1980, 139).

At the time sociologists were also beginning to explore the territory of disease and illness hitherto considered the domain of physicians. The 1950s and early 1960s in American sociology saw some pioneering work on the sociocultural aspects of health and illness. Zborowski (1952), Koos (1954), and Zola (1966) reported on how social and cultural factors influenced the perception of symptoms and health. Obviously, the sociocultural interpretation of health and illness and the experience of symptoms was in the air even in mainstream medicine, but still sociologists were not the ones called upon to rewrite the new script of American masculinity. Instead, the task fell to the psychologists, who already had an established position in the medical schools and had, through various research grants, achieved a stronger professional position than had sociologists vis-à-vis the physicians (Buck 1961).

The range for the coronary-prone personality became the preoccupation of the psychologists. In her review of the early research on Type A behavioral pattern, Virginia Price identified a theoretical vacuum in the medical research. She called for a clear theoretical framework in the field: "In fact, failure to develop a coherent conceptual model of Type A grounded in contemporary psychological theory seems to be responsible for the rather slow accumulation of generalizable and replicable empirical findings in Type A research" (Price 1982, xiii). The same view is expressed by the health psychologist Howard Friedman a decade later in an evaluation of what he calls the "atheoretical aberration" of the construct of the Type A behavioral pattern. According to Friedman, the medical focus and explicit avoidance of deeper psychosocial constructs resulted in a dead end: "The absence of a deep conceptual basis in psychological theory eventually led to confusion and sterility, as researchers became unsure as to where to turn for a more comprehensive understanding of Type A" (1990, 285). He continues, "Type B is even worse as a construct. It was defined simply as the absence of Type A characteristics. This weak conceptualization led attention away from those aspects of personality that might be healthy or protective" (1990, 285).

The psychologization of the Type A behavioral pattern began in 1965, when psychologist C. David Jenkins visited the cardiologist Meyer Friedman's research group in San Francisco and began to develop a questionnaire that would identify people with Type A behavior. Jenkins located the "coronary-prone behavior pattern" firmly in the brain: "Various clinicians and investigators have long suspected a possible pathogenetic role of the *central nervous system* in coronary heart disease (CHD), but only recently has this factor been accorded scientific scrutiny" (italics added; 1966, 599).

The instrument developed by Jenkins has been called the Jenkins Activity Survey, or JAS, questionnaire (Jenkins et al., 1979). It is a self-report instrument consisting of fifty-two multiple-choice items. A statistical analysis identified a subset of twenty-one questions that seemed to best predict Type A assessment on the basis of the Structured Interview. Its focus is on the content of the questions, rather than the behavioral response, and on self-report, rather than observation by another person (Roskies 1987, 11; Contrada et al., 1990, 647). In retrospect, Friedman himself remained skeptical of the Jenkins Activity Survey questionnaire because it was used as "an objective diagnostic instrument," rather than as a device merely to describe a certain type of behavior (Friedman and Ulmer 1984, 24). The tension between the biomedical/cardiology team and a new generation of psychologists entering the field can be noted in the chagrin Friedman expressed in his review of the history of the project: "Jenkins felt justified in writing a review [in 1971] for one of America's most conservative medical magazines [*New England Journal of Medicine*], one particularly read by thousands of physicians who treated coronary patients" (Friedman and Ulmer 1984, 24).

In the late 1960s still another measurement device was developed, the Bortner Short Rating Scale, which uses fourteen items of a semantic-differential type (Bortner 1969). The respondent is asked to locate him- or herself in the space between two opposing extremes (these measuring instruments are all reviewed in chapter 7).

There is no doubt that the cardiologists Friedman and Rosenman had ventured into a new area of research in their search for understanding the etiology of CHD. The emotional components of disease—later called the psychosocial factors influencing health—had so far been neglected in the biology-focused enterprise of post-Flexnerian American medicine.

So, what had began as a pragmatic effort by Friedman and Rosenman to spot a future cardiac patient in the office became an idea that was gradually co-opted by the psychologists and adapted to their scientific discourse. When filtered through the lens of psychology, the behavioral typing of overt behavior pattern A was transformed into Type A personality or the coronary-prone personality. While originally only the surface of Type A men had been mapped by means of behavioral typing, now there began an exploration of the interior of Type A men. It was here in the psyche itself—a man's inner life—where the cause of his failing heart resided.

At issue was more than a mere turf battle between cardiologists and psychologists. It was also a question of how both the self and health were understood in a particular historical moment and particularly of why certain activities and individual traits were defined as potential medical risk factors. To be of male gender was evidently no longer enough to fit the model of health. A man had to have a personality that did not take its toll on his health.

The health psychologists returned to an organismic theory of emotions rooted in a biological and universalistic frame of reference (Williams 1998, 122). Rather than emphasizing social class and social structure, which were pregnant in the concept of overt Type A behavior, the psychologists reintroduced an individualistic framework. This framework, captured in the concept of the Type A personality, was offered as a way of understanding the health problems of American middle-class men. Type A was a personality characterized by a set of attitudes summarized as intense ambition, competitiveness, and a chronic preoccupation with deadlines. Type A personality was a victim of the very culture and economy that had secured him his social position in the prevailing social order.

As Nikolas Rose has suggested, "Reflections upon the nature of human beings occur in all cultures and in all historical periods" (1997, 226). The rise of a new kind of self constructed as a personality emerged in American twentieth-century culture, a paradox of the era noted by Warren Susman: "Impulses that control human behavior and destiny were felt to arise more and more within the individual at the very time that the laws governing the world were seen as more and more impersonal" (1984, 272).

Susman reflects on the change of the ethical regime from men of character to men with a personality: "Thus 'personality,' like 'character,' is an effort to solve the problem of self in a changed social structure that imposes its own special demands on the self" (1984, 278; see also Rieff 1959, 356). In the United States, it was psychology as a new scientific discourse that created the modern self as an actor with his own motives: a psychological and ethical individual. The rise of psychological man indicated the emergence of a person with a certain psychological predisposition—a personality (Rieff 1959, 356).

The 1950s constituted an epoch that radically changed the conditions for American middle-class men. The transformation was imminent, although society provided a cultural setting that gave the same kind of false sense of security and tranquility as before a tornado. The decade can generally be characterized as conservative, a time of tight social and political control in which white middle-class men might at some level have sensed that their class, gender, and race supremacy was soon going to be challenged and tarnished. In this cultural, economic, and political climate, Type A man emerged as a construct to explain the problem of modern American men. Type A reflected the cultural repertoire of a set of men who shared a social position in the gender, class, and racial order. When this cultural repertoire was given a name in medical discourse—Type A—it provided a grammar for speaking of and a psychological language to reflect and express the experience of the self (Rose 1997, 235). Type A made visible a certain dimension of the self and constructed this self as an object of reflection for middle-class American men.

THE STAGES IN THE CAREER OF A MEDICAL INNOVATION

The rise and fall of the Type A thesis—the hypothesized relationship between a certain behavioral pattern and CHD—illustrates the kind of career a medical innovation has to go through before it becomes part of mainstream biomedical knowledge and standard medical practice. John McKinlay has suggested that a medical innovation generally goes through seven stages: (1) the stage of the "promising report," (2) the stage of professional and organizational adoption, (3) the stage of public acceptance and state (third-party) endorsement, (4) the stage of "standard procedure" and observational reports, (5) the stage of the randomized controlled trial (RCT), (6) the stage of professional denunciation, and (7) the stage of erosion and discreditation (1981, 375).

In the case of the Type A hypothesis, the first stage—the promising report— is represented by the seminal article in *JAMA* in 1959 by Friedman and Rosenman on Type A and the description of the six behavioral traits that characterized Type A behavioral pattern (p. 46).

The second stage—professional and organizational adoption—is represented by the application of the construct Type A as an independent variable in a number of prospective studies and the later elaboration of the concept and testing of it as Type A personality in empirical studies by health psychologists. The Framingham Heart Study represents the genre of research that applied Type A behavior as a predictor of CHD in men and women (Haynes et al., 1978a, 1978b, and 1980). In 1980, its report on the relationship of psychosocial factors to CHD stated, "Type A behavior is a significant factor for CHD in both men and women under 65 years of age" (Haynes et al., 1980, 54).

At this stage there seems to have been a conceptual wilderness in the psychological research on Type A as the psychologists tried to identify the various psychological dimensions of the Type A personality. The early research literature was murky on this issue. As Price found in her review of the indicators used in the research literature of Type A from 1959 to 1979, the characteristics associated with Type A overlapped and had not been clearly defined—for example, terms such as *aggressive*, *hostile*, *hard-driving*, *striving for achievement* appeared frequently without being properly operationalized (1982, 11–12).

The third stage—public acceptance—is represented by a number of professional reviews. In 1978, the National Heart, Lung, and Blood Institute appointed a review panel, the task of which was to evaluate available research and theory linking behavior to CHD (Review Panel on Coronary-Prone and Coronary Heart Disease 1981). At this stage there was still a consensus on the merits of the concept of Type A. In the introductory section of its report in 1981, the panel concluded, "There was general agreement that a relationship between type A behavior and CHD was supported by the data" (Review Panel on Coronary-Prone and Coronary Heart Disease 1981, 1200, also 1209). The review panel pointed, however, to a number of problems in this research. One problem was that "Incomplete understanding of mechanisms by which type A behavior influences specific disease process further hinders the assessment of its implications for health care activities" (Review Panel on Coronary-Prone and Coronary Heart Disease 1981, 1200).

Another problem centered on conceptualization and measurement. The panel was concerned about the conceptualization of Type A and noted that "confusion exists because of different terminologies, different conceptualizations and a multiplicity of measurement procedures" (Review Panel on Coronary-Prone and Coronary Heart Disease 1981, 1204). In retrospect, the methodological critique was remarkably harsh. In fact, the review panel argued that the equation of the term *coronary-prone behavior* with the Type A pattern prejudges the issue and should be abandoned (Review Panel on Coronary-Prone and Coronary Heart Disease 1981, 1209).

The fourth and fifth phases are represented by the testing of the hypothesis of Type A, an activity that grew in the 1980s. As table 4.1 shows, research on the Type A personality peaked during the period from 1985 to 1989, when almost half of all the medical literature was published.

The sixth stage—professional denunciation—started gradually to mount in the mid-1980s. For example, the hypothesis was refuted by an extensive study reported in the *New England Journal of Medicine* in 1985, which declared that "there is no uniform evidence to substantiate either a close relation between the characteristic behavior of the Type A personality and coronary disease or the protective effects of the Type B personality" (Case et al., 1985, 740). The article concluded, however, that this result did "not invalidate the effects of all emotional factors on coronary disease but suggest that more specific personality characteristics than Type A behavior need to be examined if a stronger relationship is to be defined" (Case et al., 1985, 741). The emotional component seemed to the researchers a promising area of study in future research, and they suggested, "Certain behavioral characteristics, such as

Table 4.1.   Distribution of Publications Covering "Type A Personality" as a Key Phrase, According to Medline, 1965–2002

Year	Number	Percentage
1965–1969	—	—
1970–1974	3	0.2
1975–1979	1	0.1
1980–1984	46	3.3
1985–1989	640	46.1
1990–1994	433	31.2
1995–1999	194	14.0
2000–2002	70	5.1
Total	1,387	100

Source: U.S. National Library of Medicine, Medline: PubMed (MeSH-term analysis).

hostility and unexpressed anger, may have an adverse influence on established coronary heart disease" (Case et al., 1985, 741).

A few issues later in 1985, an editorial in the *New England Journal of Medicine* stated quite bluntly that the assumption that mental state is a major factor in causing and curing specific diseases is a myth and part of folklore rather than based on scientific knowledge: "However, it is time to acknowledge that our belief in disease as a direct reflection of mental state is largely folklore. Furthermore, the corollary view of sickness and death as a personal failure is a particularly unfortunate form of blaming the victim" (Angell 1985, 1572).

Within the ranks of mainstream medicine, the critique of the relationship between Type A and CHD became more explicit, and stage seven—erosion and discreditation—was imminent. In 1988, an editorial on Type A behavior and coronary disease in the *New England Journal of Medicine* suggested that "the simple model linking Type A behavior to coronary heart disease is no longer tenable." It pointed to the controversy on the issue because of conflicting results: "Indeed, some may wonder whether the 'A' in Type A stands for 'acrimony'" (Dimsdale 1988, 110).

A whole area of research began to develop around the hypothesis that "hostility may represent the 'toxic' element of Type A behavior" (Contrada et al., 1990, 647). The negative emotional component began to be viewed as a physiologic response to environmental stressors in new biomedically oriented research in psychology and behavioral medicine (e.g., Sapolsky 1994). Research on anger, hostility, and anxiety has also continued to be pursued by a psychosomatic tradition resting on a Freudian type of assumption that repressed emotions eventually lead to illness (Friedman 1990, 5). One strand of research still clings to the personality framework, although at issue are broader emotional states. In the late 1980s, a kind of gloomy personality was coined the "generic disease-prone personality" (e.g., Friedman and Booth-Kewley 1987, 551). This disease-prone personality was quickly put in alphabetical order and redefined as a Type D, the "distressed" personality (Stone and Costa 1990, 194). In the 1990s, Type D was linked to CHD in Belgian studies (Denollet 1993, 1998, and 2000; Denollet and Van Heck 2001). Type D is, however, conceptually viewed as unrelated to Type A. As defined by its most ardent proponent, the Type D construct hypothesizes a relationship between certain personality characteristics and cardiac health: "Type D represents a personality profile characterized by both the tendency to experience negative emotions and the propensity to inhibit self-expression in social interaction" (Denollet and Van Heck 2001, 465).

The authors of a recent review of the past decades of research on personality as a coronary risk factor were quite confident that Type D represents the "toxic element" in the kind of personality type that produces coronary artery disease:

Current evidence suggests that Type D has displaced Type A as the dominant personality risk factor for coronary artery disease. Therefore to B or not to B is no longer a fitting question. Today, a more appropriate question might be, "Is there any merit in converting Type A personality to Type B, Type B to A or Type D to A or B?" (Fred and Hariharan 2002, 1)

The seventh stage—discreditation—of the Type A and Type A personality thesis is represented by the 1990s. As table 4.1 shows, a third of the research was produced between 1990 and 1994. By the mid-1990s, scant research was any longer done on the Type A thesis.

CONCLUSION

My intention in providing an overview of the fall of Type A man in this chapter has not been to validate the measures, samples, or reported results in the research on Type A behavioral pattern. This task has been conscientiously performed by representatives of mainstream medicine and epidemiology and public health, who have provided excellent overviews of the results of the genre of Type A research and the limitations of the operationalizations of the measures and of the populations studied (e.g., Keith 1966; Glass 1977; Price 1982, 13; Matthews and Haynes 1986, 926; Contrada et al., 1990; Friedman 1990; Miller et al., 1991; Hemingway and Marmot 1999). Nor has my intention been to report on how some of those limitations were addressed in later prospective studies, beginning with the Framingham Heart Study, that examined the link between psychosocial work factors or social networks or supports and heart disease (see the review by Hemingway and Marmot, 1999). Instead, my purpose has been to illustrate how suddenly at a particular time in history a certain type of masculine behavior that had been morally and financially valorized was redefined in pathological terms by mainstream medicine.

The original concept of Type A man, defined by the Type A behavioral pattern, had been an indirect critique of the other-directed character of men as part of their position in the social structure and economic production. The medical discourse on Type A had medicalized men's overt behavior and agency. The psychologization of the concept as Type A personality or the coronary-prone personality implied a penetration of men's interiors. The psychologists ventured into the interior of the middle-class man and found him to have lost his self-control, the very core of masculinity. The psychological discourse on Type A personality constructed men's emotional being as the Type A personality.

The fall of Type A man began paradoxically with the psychologization of the concept. Psychologists ventured into a new field of research as they tried to capture the various dimensions of aggression and hostility characterized early as the Type A personality. While originally a holistic and simplistic concept had been used in the medical gaze applied by the cardiologist pair Friedman and Rosenman, the creation of the Type A personality by psychological research implied a fragmentation of the concept into numerous (measurable) components. It seems that the fragmentation of Type A man into various measurable psychological components resulted in the fall of Type A man and, eventually, the fall of Type A individuals as well. Most likely the concept of a Type A personality could not serve as an equally good heuristic diagnostic device as the pioneering and holistic concept of Type A man. This fragmentation rendered Type A no longer useful as a medical discourse and the Structured Interview no longer useful as a simple diagnostic instrument for the practicing physician. The fall of the Type A man as a medical construct and distinct social and diagnostic category had begun.

Translated into the language of sociology, the medical gaze constructed, we could say, a specific male body and male psychology in medical and psychological discourse as Type A and Type A personality. This discursively inscribed male body appeared as the scientific fact of human nature: Type A was a generic individual with certain innate traits. In scientific discourse coronary-prone men were characterized by a certain behavioral pattern and personality—Type A, a type not seen as marked by gender. Type A is an example of a male body that materialized through scientific and public discourse, but remained unmarked by gender.

Nevertheless, the psychologization of Type A gave a comfortable sense that help was at hand, especially through the therapeutic work of a number of emerging personal-problems professions (Abbott 1988), an approach that R. W. Connell has called "masculinity therapy" (1987, 235). Michael A. Messner notes, "Liberated men, it seemed, could now 'get in touch with their feelings' and still feel good about their status, power and privilege over others" (1998, 265). In this sense, the psychologization of the health problems of American middle-class men was hardly surprising because this approach had a certain elective affinity to the social class in question. The psychological framework (scientific discourse) confirmed the very individualistic ethos to which these men had succumbed. A structural explanation, on the other hand, would have challenged the basic social structure—the prevailing race, class, and gendered hierarchies—that guaranteed them their privileged social position and success.

The psychologization of Type A man resulted in a shift of focus from men's overt behavior to their minds and emotions. A whole new psychology of human growth and human potential also emerged as an outgrowth of the realization of the health costs of a narrow definition of masculinity for men (e.g.,

Ehrenreich 1983, 88). The script of the traditional white middle-class man was rewritten not perhaps because this man was otherwise doomed to self-destruction, as some tend to propose (e.g., Ehrenreich 1983, 84), but perhaps to prepare him for the kind of structural changes in the labor market, the workplace, and the family that were going on or began at that time. The medicalization of Type A man was the first effort in modern etiological thinking that addressed the health costs of traditional masculinity and suggested that men adopt a more relaxed and healthy lifestyle in order to stay healthy (Ehrenreich 1983, 84). In sociological terms it meant that men could be resocialized and thereby adopt a "healthier" male identity.

In retrospect, perhaps the mythology of the Type A man—the core of which was the coronary-prone personality—was the grand narrative and the essential image that was needed for these men to turn to a healthy lifestyle previously connected more with the rules governing the behavior of women than that of "real" men. As others have suggested, masculinities have long been defined against a healthy lifestyle—so-called positive health behaviors (see also Berrett 1997; Courtenay 2000). The traditional medical risk factors (smoking, hypertension, physical inactivity), embraced by the pre– and post–Type A man epidemiologists, alerted Type A men to the unhealthy life they were living in a consumerist society. This biomedical epidemiological paradigm had all along suggested that certain behaviors, like smoking, being sedentary, and eating fatty foods, not a certain personality, were the real culprits in the rising CHD rates among middle-class men. In fact, in 1968—in the heyday of the Type A thesis—a surprising epidemiological turn took place: CHD mortality rates began to decline in the United States. Between 1968 and 1976, the rates declined by 21 percent, and it has been estimated that about half (54 percent) of the decline in cardiovascular mortality rates can be attributed to changes in lifestyle during this period (Goldman and Cook 1984, 825).

Type A man and the coronary-prone personality were powerful representations of the plight of the middle-class man, images that became part of the medical folklore and popular discourse of the American middle class. Type A constituted a central concept in the vocabulary of a cohort of the American population in the 1960s and 1970s, whose consciousness about work was formed by the notions of the behavioral pattern of a Type A person. For this generation, Type A was an idiom for marking career-oriented individuals: they were Type A. Type A was not only a marker, but also a lens through which individuals could analyze the emotional and physical costs involved in the modern organization of work. White-collar work demanded a commitment and work ethic of its workers, a moral dimension of work previously the hallmark of the small entrepreneur. But more importantly, it was no longer the medical profession, but instead laypeople, who began to diagnose themselves as Type A. Equipped with a new psychological gaze, they were able to define, reflect upon, and communicate to others their own work ambitions and the health costs of this ambition. As Rose has suggested, the field of psychology has been an essential framework for constructing the modern self: "We can experience ourselves as certain types of creatures only because we do so under a certain description" (1997, 234). Type A became such a label of the modern self. To state, "I am a Type A," has been a way of positioning oneself in the moral order and in the social hierarchy of work. In this hierarchy the centrality of work and the work ethic has dominated and defined the moral individual. It is in this sense that Type A has served as a marker in the construction, in the words of Michèle Lamont, of the moral boundaries between social classes of men in the labor force (1992 and 2000).

Chapter Five

How the Hardy Executive Supplanted Type A Man

As chapters 3 and 4 showed, in the beginning of the 1950s and through the subsequent three decades, there was an earnest effort to understand the new cultural syndrome of "stress," so prevalent in the post–World War II, work-oriented world. This syndrome became the concern of the North American medical community, which undertook to explore its complex character.

The medical literature saw the health problems of Type A men in behavioral and psychological terms: the behavioral style and the psychological disposition of certain men made them prone to heart disease. Yet, these behaviors and psychological traits were not randomly distributed. On the contrary, they were predominantly found among white middle-class, middle-aged men, Type A men. Nevertheless, the early studies on Type A were not based on a random sample of individuals. Instead, Type A behavior was studied among groups of employed middle-class American men selected because they worked in a certain occupation and work setting (a group identified as having a high prevalence of CHD). For example, about 80 percent of the men included in the pioneering follow-up study called the Western Collaborative Group Study, conducted by Rosenman and his colleagues (1975) were employed in white-collar occupations (see Haynes et al., 1980, 55).

But as chapter 4 shows, Type A as a diagnostic category began to lose its predictive power and scientific relevance by the mid-1980s. By this time, a new construct entered medical knowledge via health psychology, a personality disposition called "hardiness."

This chapter describes the transition in the stress literature from a focus on Type A man to the "hardy executive." I show how these concepts were constructed and translated in medical and psychological discourse and that they related to notions of masculinity, class, and health. With the aid of a new construct—hardiness—the transition of middle-class men from unhealthy

Type A men to hardy and healthy could be explained. At the same time, hardiness added legitimacy to the core values of middle-class masculinity. In more sociological terms, hardiness became a key to reevaluating the traditional version of the male role and reinventing the core features of what Pleck has called the modern version of the male sex role (1976, 156–157). The concept of the hardy executive suggested a new relationship between men's attitudes, work behavior, and health.

HOW THE HARDY EXECUTIVE SUPPLANTED TYPE A MAN

In the late 1970s a new discourse was introduced in health psychology that identified a personality predisposition called hardiness. This disposition is assumed to protect men from the deleterious effects of stress on their health. It is assumed that a new generation of middle-class men can look forward to a new relationship between their social position and health: men can be ambitious, compete, be in control, succeed, and still be healthy. In contrast to Type A man, driven by a seemingly irrational passion to reach extrinsic goals and rewards, the hardy man is constructed as one who is driven by primarily intrinsic motivation. Both personality structures seem to emphasize drive, involvement, and goal striving.

The latter construct—hardiness—was introduced in 1979 by Suzanne Kobasa, who developed it further in a couple of subsequent articles (Kobasa et al., 1981, 1982, and 1983) and in a book *The Hardy Executive* (Maddi and Kobasa 1984). According to Kobasa, hardiness is a personality characteristic: "Persons who experience high degrees of stress without falling ill have a personality structure differentiating them from persons who become sick under stress" (1979, 3). Kobasa views "hardy persons" as sharing three characteristics: control, commitment, and a sense that change is a personal challenge. By possessing these characteristics, a hardy person is able to remain healthy under stress, while "the highly stressed persons who become ill are powerless, nihilistic, and low in motivation for achievement" (Kobasa 1979, 3).

To test the effect of hardiness, Kobasa examined a group of middle- and upper-level executives ($n = 670$) of a large public utility company, a homogeneous group selected so that all were males, forty to forty-nine years old, married with two children, wife not working outside the home, usually Protestant, and attending religious services very or fairly often (Kobasa 1979, 5). The study aimed at exploring "the importance of personality as a conditioner of the illness-provoking effects of stress" (Kobasa 1979, 1). Kobasa's hypotheses about hardiness were confirmed. She concludes, "The mechanism whereby stressful life events produce illness is presumably physiological. Whatever this physiological response is, the personality characteristics of hardiness may cut into it, decreasing the likelihood of breakdown into illness" (Kobasa 1979, 9).

In the discussion about the findings, Kobasa constructs a hypothetical hardy executive who has to deal with a job transfer (1979, 9). The transfer is not envisioned as a threat for the hardy man, but experienced as a challenge: "The hardy executive does more than passively acquiesce to the job transfer" (Kobasa 1979, 9). The positive attitude allows the hypothetical executive to throw "himself actively into the new situation, utilizing his inner resources to make it his own." And Kobasa portrays the hardy executive and his less hardy counterpart in the following terms:

> An *internal* (rather than *external*) locus of control allows the hardy executive to greet the transfer with the recognition that although it may have been initiated in an office above him, the actual course it takes is dependent upon how he handles it. For all these reasons, he is not just a victim of a threatening change but an active determinant of the consequences it brings about. In contrast, the executive low in hardiness will react to the transfer with less sense of personal resource, more acquiescence, more encroachments of meaninglessness, and a conviction that change has been externally determined with no possibility of control on his part. In this context, it is understandable that the hardy executive will also tend to perceive the transfer as less personally stressful than his less hardy counterpart. (1979, 9)

In contrast to Type A man, the hardy executive is characterized by self-control, the very core of traditional masculine identity. The challenges awaiting the executive—whether hardy or not—are "learning to cope with new subordinates and supervisors, finding a new home, helping children and wife with a new school and neighborhood" (Kobasa 1979, 5).

A later prospective study of white, married, middle- and upper-level male executives ($n = 259$) of a large utility company followed this group for five years and tested the effects of the "hardy personality style" on their health. This personality style is characterized as follows: "Hardy persons have considerable curiosity and tend to find their experiences interesting and meaningful. Further, they believe they can be influential through what they imagine, say, and do. At the same time they expect change to be the norm, and regard it as an important stimulus to development" (Kobasa et al., 1981, 368). In contrast, "persons low in hardiness tend to find themselves and their environment boring, meaningless, and threatening. They feel powerless in the face of overwhelming forces, believing that life is best when it involves no changes" (Kobasa et al., 1981, 369).

As a consequence of the lack of hardiness, "because their personalities provide little or no buffer, the stressful events are allowed to have a debilitating effect on health." This and a later study of the same group both confirm the hypothesis that "hardiness is a constellation of personality characteristics that function as a resistance resource in the encounter with stressful life events" (Kobasa et al., 1982, 169, see also 1981 and 1983; Ouelette 1993). Although Kobasa in the first part of her presentation of the construct of hardiness only uses the terms *hardy personality*, *hardy persons*, and *hardy individuals*, both her sample of males and her example of the hardy executive indicate that the concept in question is male gendered.

THE HARDY EXECUTIVE

The hardy executive is the focus of an incisive gaze in *The Hardy Executive: Health under Stress* (1984), in which Salvatore Maddi and Suzanne Kobasa summarize the findings reported in their previously published scientific articles (e.g., Kobasa et al., 1981 and 1982). In more popular language and in greater detail, the book provides an overview of the background, methodology, and findings of their study of a group of 259 middle- and upper-level executives in a company, Illinois Bell. In addressing the question of why personality hardiness makes a difference for whether or not a person becomes ill in the face of stress, Maddi and Kobasa in the introductory chapter present the vignettes of the lives of four men: Chuck and Bill, who are both high in hardiness, and Jim and Andy, who are both low in hardiness. Chuck and Bill display commitment through their interest in their work, family, and friends. By being "in control," they are influential, it is suggested, in all three spheres. In contrast, Jim and Andy feel lonely, bored, displaced, powerless, and vulnerable. The lesson learned is that the first two can handle stress, while the latter two cannot cope with it.

For Maddi and Kobasa, hardiness is a personality style that evolves around "The BIG 3": commitment rather than alienation, control rather than powerlessness, and challenge rather than threat (1984, 31). These characteristics, the reader is told, are molded during childhood because a certain "family atmosphere breeds hardiness." Supportive parents are assumed to encourage their children to have a sense of mastery. As Maddi and Kobasa phrase it, "In this atmosphere, youngsters are very likely to develop hardiness, taking it with them as they become older and leave their families" (1984, 50).

Maddi and Kobasa argue in fact that the values underlying the primary (gender) socialization are more important in breeding hardiness than are the material conditions. They suggest that "atmosphere is something established for children by their parents, and it bears little or no relationship to economic and social advantage or disadvantage" (1984, 52). Nevertheless, hardiness, they note, can be learned at any time in life, and an executive can turn to "counseling for hardiness" (which is the title of chapter 6 of their book). With the aid of counseling, certain self-management techniques can be inculcated (techniques that Foucault [1988] would have called technologies of the self). From a sociological perspective, the authors seem to suggest that the qualities of hardiness can be acquired through proper resocialization of the male executive. Men can acquire a refurbished healthy male identity required for a successful managerial performance in working life.

But there is more than the mere question of personal control at stake. In addition to fostering their own health, hardy executives have economic advantages for the company. Hardiness, it is suggested, is a personality disposition that it is in the interest of the company to promote among its executives because "health influences productivity, and this translates directly into profitability," and "it makes sense, therefore, for companies to foster hardiness in their employees" (Maddi and Kobasa 1984, 76). Maddi and Kobasa conclude, "Hardy executives are especially effective because they are not passively compliant. This is yet another way in which hardiness seems to contribute to profitability" (1984, 78).

And in harder times when the company faces the consequences of structural and economic change, Maddi and Kobasa write "While nonhardy executives shrug their shoulders in the face of the recession and unemployment, for example, hardy managers are probably looking for ways of making the best of a difficult situation" (1984, 92).

As the above quotations show, the hardy man is a type who has character and is therefore able to withstand changes in the workplace. Type A man responded to the comparable institutional dilemma in the 1950s with hostility, aggression, a sense of powerlessness, and lack of control in the face of changes in the conditions of work and concomitant perceived threats to his male role and identity. Type A man captured the enigma of the white-collar man in the 1950s as described by C. Wright Mills: "He is pushed by forces beyond his control, pulled into movements he does not understand; he gets into situations in which his is the most helpless position. The white-collar man is the hero as victim" (1951, xii).

In contrast, the hardy man faces the institutional dilemmas equipped with different attitudes and behaviors. His major strength is that he is not extrinsically, but intrinsically, motivated in his work and personal life. Although he is success-oriented like Type A, the hardy executive is responsible, actively coping with challenges and changes in his economic and social surroundings. The hardy executive endures the challenges of the flexibility and uncertainty that characterize the workplace and the labor market in a post-Fordist economy. His achievements are related to his interpersonal and problem-solving skills, which enable him to pursue the goals he is committed to.

The hardy executive seems to have the kind of character that Richard Sennett thought the prevailing capitalism had corroded (1998). The hardy man emerges as a refurbished representation of the moral foundation of entrepreneurial capitalism, a spirit assumed to result in wealth and the public good. The hardy executive captures the individual responsibility of the classic Weberian spirit of capitalism, to which even President George W. Bush alluded in his talk to Wall Street financiers in New York on July 9, 2002, when he commented on the financial scandals surrounding Enron and WorldCom (2002). A resurrection of the spirit of individual responsibility is needed, Bush said, calling for a "new ethic of personal responsibility" in the business community, because "lasting wealth and prosperity are built on a foundation of integrity." "In the long run," Bush said, "there is no capitalism without conscience; there is no wealth without character." The remedy for the ailing American corporate community is to revitalize the spirit of capitalism and its moral foundation; the reformed capitalist spirit would heal the American economy: "We need men and women of character who know the difference between ambition and destructive greed, between justified risk and irresponsibility, between enterprise and fraud" (Bush 2002). It seems as if the hardy executive is up to the moral demands set in the president's Wall Street address. The hardy executive embodies the Protestant ethic and the spirit of capitalism—the psychological conditions that make possible the development and success of a capitalist economy (see Weber 1958).

MEDICALIZATION AND DEMEDICALIZATION OF MASCULINITY

The term hardiness has become an established concept in health psychology research. From 1979 to 2000, of the 296 articles listed under the key word "hardiness" in a Medline search, 225 are on hardiness as a health-protective factor (U.S. National Library of Medicine 2003) (the rest of the articles chiefly deal with disease-resistant plants, insects, and organisms).

During the first five years, the research mainly studied white middle-class, middle-aged men, as had the early research on Type A man. But ten years after the introduction of the concept of hardiness, it is used in portraying the personality characteristics of those who can cope with stressful circumstances: how patients with chronic disease cope with illness or how people subject to serious stress cope with their lives. An interesting genre, related to the latter theme, has been research on nurses and their coping with work stress and burnout. Since 1985, this theme appears frequently in articles published in nursing journals (e.g., McCranie et al., 1987; Simoni and Paterson 1997; see Riska and Wrede 2003).

Type A and hardiness are central concepts in a scientific discourse that aims to explain differences in health by making personality a risk factor for illness. Although in focus are relatively fixed personality characteristics and individual traits, both psychological categories describe a group of men sharing certain social positions in the economic and gender order. The personality — whether Type A personality or the hardy personality — is conceptualized as the type of masculinity that relates to the health of the American middle class. The medical risk factor of Type A man seems to be his overconformity to the work ethic: while he conforms to the ideal of achievement and hard work, he is not in control of his own life. Type A is characterized by aggressive and impulsive behavior, and he has poor interpersonal skills. By contrast, the hardy man is also achievement oriented, but he looks forward to his promotion and social mobility because he has a sense of self-control and purpose. He has the interpersonal skills expected of modern managers, and he remains emotionally constrained — self-disciplined — even in hard situations. Yet, as cultural idioms of respective decades — the 1950s and 1980s — the two psychological categories capture the inner life of the two types of men who were the crucial economic actors of their society. They also capture the constraints and opportunities — both in economic and cultural terms — of these men during the respective decades. While the construct of Type A man medicalized traditional masculinity, the construct of hardiness redefines and reinvents masculinity for modern middle-class men. Men are now told that they can be committed to the American work ethic without having to pay the health costs for this kind of behavior, if they can remain in control and be responsible.

The construct of hardiness not only demedicalizes certain economic and social behavior, but more importantly, it legitimizes a new view of masculinity. Men can now have a comfortable sense of mastery of their stress levels or rationalize that stress might even be good for them. Yet, what the new construct of hardiness did was to confirm that hard work, autonomy, and self-control are core virtues of middle-class masculinity.

But both representations — Type A man and the hardy man — individualize differences in health, although the concepts are based on social categories, especially the social positions of class and gender. The concept of hardiness diffuses the social character of masculinity: Masculine behavior is captured as an individual characteristic and personality disposition, rather than an institution and a set of structures that privilege a certain type of white middle-class male behavior. It is in this sense that the Type A man and the hardy man are more than mere categories of individual identities. They capture the tacit power relations and hidden hierarchies of super- and subordination based on class, race, and gender.

A broader understanding of these men's health would have been achieved if the social contextual factors had been recognized. Such an analysis would have revealed a social patterning of health and the link between social conditions and individual well-being. For example, the early research on Type A man and on hardiness was conducted with white middle-class men (see Funk and Houston 1987; Funk 1992). While Type A men were selected by social class and recruited from mainly executive positions and commitment to traditional masculinity as a trait, so were those examined for hardiness. Type A men were selected for subgroup A compared to group B and group C on the basis of expressed masculinity as an overt individual behavioral style. Similarly, hardy executives were selected on the basis of social class and an overt behavior fitting traditional heterosexual masculinity: They were selected because they conformed to the nuclear-family pattern and male-breadwinner ideal (see p. 60).

As a representation, hardiness is a gentrified version of the populist spirit of the hard and self-made man. Hardness has been a central feature of American (male) mythology, in which rugged individualism and physical strength have shaped the self-made man of both agrarian and white-collar stripe (see Hofstadter 1955; Kimmel 1997). The next section examines a special cultural genre in American popular culture, the Hardy Boys books. The Hardy Boys series set the stage for a gentrified version of hardness and constructed hardiness as an ideal for modern American males. The Hardy Boys series could be seen as a cultural production that presages the emergence of the hardy man.

HARDINESS IN POPULAR DISCOURSE

The cultural production of self-control and mastery as the revered ideal for the American man has a long history in American popular discourse, as shown in Michael Kimmel's 1997 review of the cultural history of manhood in America. Kimmel's analysis focuses on the cultural construction of the self-made man. Another recent cultural analysis of the construction of the American male as an object of idealization and cultural consumption by Susan Bordo supports Kimmel's portrayal, but Bordo's analysis lacks the incisive links to structures of power found in Kimmel's work (2000). Neither Kimmel nor Bordo mentions one genre of cultural production of the masculine in the twentieth century: the Hardy Boys. Introduced in 1927, this was a series of mystery stories for boys. These books told the adventures of Joe and Frank Hardy—brothers with hardy spirits, amateur sleuths who were great problem solvers (McFarlane 1976; Billman 1986; Johnson 1993). Revised versions of these stories were republished by Simon and Schuster in the early 1980s when, incidentally, the hardy man was introduced in health psychology. The small-town context and problem-solving capacities of the Hardy boys and the hardy executive constitute an interesting common denominator.

The Hardy Boys: A Theme Is Born in American Mythology

The Hardy Boys was not the first series of mystery stories for boys in the United States. The Rover Boys series was introduced in 1899 and ran until 1926, and the Tom Swift series was on the market from 1910 to 1941. Neither of these managed to capture the imagination as the Hardy Boys did, or to achieve their sales figures. The Hardy Boys in many respects represented a new literary genre. The books were produced by Edward Stratemeyer, who employed ghostwriters in his publishing empire for most of the series. The Hardy Boys books were mass-produced and became "a Henry Ford of fiction for boys and girls," as the genre has been characterized by Leslie McFarlane, the writer of most of them (1976, 9). The Hardy Boys offered an armchair opportunity for consuming adventures for a pre-television-age generation of teenagers who inhabited a world in which juvenile leisure was becoming an economic and cultural option. Previous series of boys' books had been about boys confronting adventures in exotic and almost unreal conditions. The Hardy Boys introduced a new and enormously successful setting in American cultural consumption: the peaceful small town that provides a safe and familiar setting for adventures. This genre shows that adventure can be found in a sleeping and seemingly static American town, where the problems and exotic features of the outside world come to and confront you in your own back yard. This makes the stories not only plausible, but also surprisingly scary. This theme has, for example, later been picked up by Steven Spielberg in his movie production—the movie *ET* perhaps best captures this cultural imagery.

The principal writer of the Hardy Boys books, Leslie McFarlane, alias Franklin W. Dixon, was a Canadian who started as a small-town journalist, but became the ghostwriter of the series from 1927 to 1946. "I probably had a knack for storytelling," he reminisces, "the entertainer's gift which can always be polished to the glow of art" (McFarlane 1976, 187). The introduction of two brothers was another new and successful theme. As McFarlane notes, "Two heroes were better than one, because they always had someone to talk to and they could take turns in being rescuer and rescuee" (1976, 198). Compared to the detective fiction written for an adult audience, like that by Dashiell Hammett and Raymond Chandler, the Hardy Boys books were moral and sanitized of any rough language and insinuation of interest in girls or women. As McFarlane himself confesses about the construction of the moral profile of the Hardy boys, "Literature these books were not but, by God, they were Moral! You could fault them on any grounds you liked, but never on turpitude!" (1976, 178).

The Hardy boys—Frank, who is 16, and Joe, who is 15—live at home with their father and mother and go to high school in a fictitious small town, Bayport, on Barmet Bay, somewhere on the Atlantic coast. The small-town setting provides a community frozen in time, just as the Hardy boys are frozen characters and perennial teenagers. As Carol Billman, a commentator on the series, notes, "It is a frozen and fixed world where mysteries come and go, but there is no change or human complexity" (1986, 93). Another commentator on the Hardy Boys and on a later but equally popular series for girls, Nancy Drew, reflects on Bayport on the East Coast and River Heights in the Midwest: "The real world stops at the edges of both towns, where no citizens suffer from the Great Depression, are called to fight in any war, or have reason to protest social injustice" (Kismaric and Heiferman 1998, 52).

The Hardy family is a full-fledged nuclear family. The father of the boys, Fenton Hardy, now forty years old, has his own detective practice after being on the New York police force. The boys' mother, Laura Hardy, is a traditional housewife who occasionally appears from the kitchen as a provider of food for the family and for the boys' friends. The father serves as a powerful male role model for his sons, who aspire to become detectives when they grow up. In the opening sentence of the first volume, *The Tower Treasure,* the boys ponder their transition from adolescence to the adult world of men and a future of being detectives. They valorize the role model of their father: "Why shouldn't we? Isn't he one of the most famous detectives in the country? And aren't we his sons? If the profession was good for him to follow it should be good enough for us" (Dixon 1927, 1). "Nothing offered so many possibilities of adventure and excitement as the career of a detective" (Dixon 1927, 3).

The father tacitly supports the career choice of the boys, while the mother has other plans for securing her sons' middle-class status. As one of the brothers laments, "She comes out plump and plain and says she wants one of us to be a doctor and the other a lawyer" (Dixon 1927, 3). But the boys are dreaming of getting "a mystery all of our own to solve one day," because as Joe Hardy exclaims, "if we do we'll show that Fenton Hardy's sons are worthy of his name. Oh boy, but what wouldn't I give to be famous as Dad!" (Dixon 1927, 4). Their dreams are soon fulfilled when their own first case is introduced in *The Tower Treasure,* where the rest of their high school friends are also presented to the readers. This group of boys is surprisingly diverse in social class and ethnicity. Theirs is a world untroubled by people of female gender and by emotions, a circumstance that leaves them free to explore the world of action and to protect the peace and safety of their small town (Kismaric and Heiferman 1998, 36). Kismaric and Heiferman reflect on the cultural image of the Hardy boys: "They simply affirm their loyalties, believe in their own invulnerability and unwavering moral strength, and act out their version of masculinity in a timeless, endless hoop of thrilling excitements" (1998, 46).

Fenton Hardy, the father, is an internationally famous detective, a profession he characterizes this way: "In my business I have to take chances" (Dixon 1928, 22). As often as he assists and introduces his sons to the art of detective work and its spirit of professionalism, the boys provide crucial help in solving their father's cases (e.g., in the fourth volume, *The Missing Chums* [Dixon 1928]). The Hardy boys also take chances, but they always get away from the tight grip of crooks or dangerous places because they are *hardy* boys, and they work perfectly as a team.

The series was produced for over half a century. The original ghostwriter, McFarlane, wrote his last book, *The Phantom Freighter*, in 1946, but the series continued long after that. McFarlane, with some chagrin, reflects on his retirement from being the first ghostwriter of the series: "The world had changed for the Hardy Boys as it had for everyone else. It is a very strange world indeed, when a ghost could be dispossessed by another ghost" (1976, 210). As the years have passed, the original external image of the Hardy boys as dressed in suit, necktie, and hat (see, for example, the pictures of the inner cover of *The Tower Treasure* [1927] and *The Phantom Freighter* [1947]) has changed to more casual dress. But the moral purity of the boys has become even more stringent—they became even more hardy and moral over the years. The mockery of the local police force and lack of respect for institutions that appeared in the early volumes were McFarlane's trademark. These features were pruned from later editions. McFarlane never consented to this purification and resented the revisions: "Even a ghost has feelings like anyone else" (1976, 211).

The Reinvention of Character

When medicine adopted the idea that Type A personality was an explanation for the development of CHD among a certain group of men, it reflected the larger visions of self and society. In the 1950s, Americans had come to be obsessed by an interest in the performance of the self. *Personality* was a term that captured the vision of self striving toward self-fulfillment, self-expression, and self-confidence, features needed in a consumer-oriented society. These hedonistic traits contrasted with the qualities of "the moral athlete of Protestant culture" in the nineteenth and early twentieth centuries, the signifier of which was "character" (Rieff 1959, 356; Susman 1984, 273).

When hardiness was introduced into the medical vocabulary in the early 1980s, the change in terminology also suggested a broader cultural shift in the kind of traits envisioned as needed for success in a new social and cultural order. The cultural shift signaled the reimagination of the meanings of dominant masculinity. The reimagination reinvented character, a classical theme in

American popular discourse, as shown in the Hardy Boys series. It was no longer hardness, but rather its gentrified version, hardiness, that was privileged. The valorization of hardiness rests on shared features between the Hardy boys and the hardy executive. These features could be called commitment, control, challenge—the three core dimensions of the construct of hardiness developed by Maddi and Kobasa (1984, 31).

First, the Hardy boys and the hardy executive are committed to their family, friends, and small-town life. The nuclear-family ideology is a given and the broader cultural matrix within which they find their own self-confidence and identity as men.

Second, the Hardy boys and the hardy executive are action oriented. Theirs is a world of full agency. They have clear goals and adopt a problem-solving approach to life and its challenges. Although they act fast and encounter difficult situations, they never lose self-control because they are committed to certain ideals.

Third, they accept whatever challenge confronts them in their everyday life, because challenges in life are personal challenges and like adventures in that they provide an opportunity for an exploration of the self and the search for and validation of male identity. Yet, these boys and men are team players and show social responsibility. In short, the Hardy boys and the hardy executive have character, that moral fiber that makes them never give up, makes them work hard, makes them work for the public interest instead of their own self-interest.

CONCLUSION

This chapter has shown that health psychology identified men's health, especially that of the gendered and embodied man in research on men's health, and integrated this insight into a new construct of hardiness. The narrow focus on individual personality structures did not do justice to the more profound revelation of the link between social structure and biography (Mills 1951 and 1959): Type A personality and the hardy personality are not merely characteristics of individuals, but social characters shaped by a social milieu. The psychological categories of Type A man and hardy man used by American medicine and health psychology have in fact indirectly suggested that stress and health inequality are related to men's positions in the gender order and in the social hierarchy at work.

In contrast to Type A, hardiness has not become a key concept in medical discourse, nor is it explicitly connected to heart disease. Instead, it is a state of psychological well-being that acts as a stress-resistant factor and as a factor in resistance to chronic disease for the very same social category of men—white middle-class executives—as described in the discourse on Type A.

In many ways, the scientific discourse in medicine and psychology on Type A has been a historical prerequisite for the later "stress research"—more lately, burnout and distress—as the pathogenic reason for a variety of chronic diseases. While Type A has captured the disease-promoting features of a certain behavioral and personality-based style, the construct of hardiness was the beginning of a new genre of research that began to look at the health-promoting features of a certain disposition. From the perspective of men's health, we could summarize the consequences in the following way: to be a Type A man has serious health costs and is an "unhealthy" male identity, while the hardy man represents a health-promoting trait and a "healthy" male identity.

In terms of the Foucauldian framework used in the analysis of the personality types, hardiness represents a discursive subject who is able to discipline and manage his or her body through self-control. According to Rose, the skills of self-direction and self-management are central features of American working life, which privileges the goals of self-actualization and individual success through the marketplace (1999, 117).

At a cultural level the construct of hardiness has recaptured the key values of American male mythology: the idealized image of hardness in American men. Hardness and self-discipline have been central features of the cultural production of maleness in books, movies, and TV series in post–World War II America (Kimmel 1997; Bordo 2000). Hardiness is a gentrified representation of hardness, an imagery in public discourse that was constructed in the Hardy Boys series. The enormous popularity of the Hardy Boys came to presage the ethical regime of hardiness in the cohort of ten-year-old readers of those books in the 1940s and 1950s. By the late 1970s, these readers were middle-aged men who had entered the career ladder of the labor force. In the early 1980s, when the theme of hardiness was introduced in psychological discourse, it resonated with the cultural heritage of an era of readers of Hardy Boys books. This cultural heritage is transmitted to the twenty-first century via a Hardy Boys lifestyle manual. In 2002, the publishers of the Hardy Boys issued a condensed package of the life wisdom and spirit of the boys: *The Hardy Boys Guide to Life* (Dixon 2002). The book contains one-to-two-sentence excerpts from the major classics of the series. The jacket promises that the Hardy boys can teach you how to master most situations: "Because the Hardy boys know what it's like to be in the heart of the action, and they always manage to find a way out of the stickiest of jams."

Chapter Six

John Henryism: The Hard-Working Marginal Man

CORONARY HEART DISEASE IN BLACKS: AN UNDERRESEARCHED ISSUE

About thirty years after the introduction of Type A, African American men entered the scientific discourse of health psychology literature when a new psychological trait was conceived: John Henryism. This term was constructed to explain the coronary health of African American men, whose health had now become of interest to researchers.

A number of reasons can be mentioned for the surge in research into the health of African Americans, some sociopolitical, some epidemiological. The sociopolitical reasons harken back to the social reform efforts initiated in the mid-1960s as part of the war on poverty and the community programs under the auspices of the Office of Economic Opportunity (OEO), notably the Community Action Program (CAP) in 1964, which called for the involvement of local residents in the implementation of services. The participation of the poor was encouraged by the slogan "maximum feasible participation," which was a way to encourage the poor, often a synonym for blacks, to be involved in the inner-city programs sponsored through federal funding (Rose 1972).[1]

The ill health of the poor was interpreted as reflecting a lack of or poor access to health services. The establishment of community mental-health and neighborhood health centers in the late 1960s in poor areas was an effort to improve access to local health services, although Krause has provocatively argued that these centers mainly advanced the careers of a "new wave" of community-oriented academic-medicine professionals, rather than met the needs of the poor (1973, 454; see also Rose 1972). Others have pointed to the initiatives of political activists who promoted the health needs of blacks and other minorities in the establishment of community clinics for underserved groups in the 1960s and 1970s (Waitzkin 2000; Sardell 1988). The gains achieved in the health of blacks, in their access to health services, and in their representation in the medical profession during the period from 1965 and 1975 have been the reason for calling this era the "Second Reconstruction" (Byrd and Clayton 2002, 575). The comparable health statistics for blacks after 1980 show a halt in the positive development or even, in some areas, a negative trend.

A more recent market-driven reason for the interest in the health of blacks is the rise of a black middle class that, comprising consumers of health care, constitutes a new market and a group with new consumer needs.

A sociopolitical reason for the focus on the health of African Americans is the public disclosure of the racism inherent in the structure of the American health care system and in American medicine (Byrd and Clayton 2002, 417–476). The result has been the establishment of rules to protect human subjects in biomedical research and to set clear ethical standards in medical research. An example was the revelation and unfolding of the Tuskegee Syphilis Study conducted by the United States Public Health Service over forty years (1932–1972) to trace the "natural history" of untreated syphilis on adult African American rural men (a total of 399 African American men were diagnosed positive for latent syphilis and studied for as long as the study went on, but they were never informed of the lack of treatment). The medical historian Allan Brandt has suggested that the study revealed more about the pathology of racism than it did about the pathology of syphilis (2000, 29). As he notes, the experiment was widely reported in mainstream medicine for forty years without evoking any significant protest within the medical community. The history of the Tuskegee Syphilis Study was finally given public closure in a formal apology presented by President Bill Clinton in a White House ceremony in 1997 (Reverby 2000).

The epidemiological reasons are grounded in the early findings on the prevalence of CHD and the rates of CHD mortality in blacks and whites. The early prospective studies on Type A and CHD, such as the Western Collaborative Group Study and the Framingham Heart Study, were done on white subjects, whose health was thought to presage the universal pattern for CHD in modern society. The tacit assumption was that the risk factors were the same for blacks. This assumption was soon challenged by new data.

Two prospective cohort studies were initiated in the southeastern United States in 1960—the Charleston Heart Study and the Evans County, Georgia, Heart Study—with the purpose of identifying risk factors for CHD in blacks and whites. The studies presented three major findings, which became the focus of debate and research during subsequent decades. First, the prevalence rates for CHD were higher for the Charleston than the Evans County study, a finding indicating that, even for blacks, the rates were higher in urban than in rural areas. Second, the prevalence of CHD was markedly lower in blacks than in whites, although hypertension—a risk factor for CHD—was twice as prevalent among blacks. Third, there was a marked difference between the CHD rates of white and black men, but no difference between the rates of black and white women (e.g., Keil and Saunders 1991; Keil et al., 1991).

Later studies on CHD mortality continued to document higher rates in whites than in blacks (Keil et al., 1984, 1993, and 1995), but other studies showed higher rates in blacks (Gillum and Liu 1984; Barnett et al., 1999; Corti et al., 1999). The latter finding is confirmed in today's national health statistics on death rates from CHD published by the National Center for Health Statistics (U.S./NCHS 2003, 32–33). As table 6.1 shows, today black males die of heart disease at the rate of 407.8 per 100,000 resident population, while white males die at a rate of 332.2 per 100,000 resident population.

Three other observations can be made from table 6.1. First, from 1950 to 1970, white males had higher death rates from heart diseases than black males, but since 1980 black males have had higher death rates from heart diseases than have white males. For blacks these rates most likely reflect gradual access to health services and to hospitals because integration into a social organization of health care is a prerequisite for the coding of the incidence, prevalence, and death rates of heart disease.

Second, women had lower rates than men regardless of race during the period from 1950 through 1998, but it is important to note that since 1950, black women have consistently had higher rates than white women. Black men have certainly had higher death rates from heart diseases than black women,

Table 6.1. Age-Adjusted Death Rates for Diseases of the Heart by Sex and Race, United States, 1950–1998*

Sex and Race	1950	1960	1970	1980	1990	1998	Change from 1950 to 1998 (%)
Male							
White	700.2	694.5	640.2	539.6	409.2	333.2	−52
Black	639.4	615.2	607.3	561.4	485.4	407.8	−36
Female							
White	478.0	441.7	376.7	315.9	250.9	217.6	−54
Black	536.9	488.9	435.6	378.6	327.5	291.9	−46
All people[†]	586.8	559.0	492.7	412.1	321.8	272.4	−54

Source: U.S. National Center for Health Statistics, 2003, Table 37.
* Rates are deaths per 100,000 resident population. Data are based on death certificates.
[†] These rates include other racial and ethnic groups.

but still it has been black men's death rates from heart diseases rather than black women's high rate vis-à-vis white women that have generated a need to develop interventions and new research instruments to understand coronary disease in blacks.

Third, the death rate has in all gender and race groups been continuously declining, especially since 1970. This decline is made more visible in table 6.1, which converts the declining rates into percentages. For example, from 1950 to 1998, the death rate from heart disease abated by 52 percent among white males, but only by 36 percent among black males, a health gap that has persisted until more recently. During the past two decades, the death rate from heart diseases declined by 38 percent among white males, but only by 27 percent among black males. Women's death rates have not fared as well as men's (31 percent decline among white women, and 21 percent among black women).

There was an inherent paradox in the early findings related to CHD in blacks: many of the known CHD risk factors (i.e., hypertension, cigarette smoking among males, obesity among females) were more prevalent in blacks than in whites, and researchers asked why CHD morbidity and mortality rates were not considerably higher in blacks than in whites (e.g., James 1984a, 669). The higher prevalence of high blood pressure and hypertension in the African American population was not only puzzling, but a reason for medical concern. In addition, psychosocial factors have been assumed to play a major role as a risk factor also for CHD in black populations (e.g., Kumanyika and Adams-Campbell 1991). Nevertheless, past instruments for measuring psychosocial factors had been developed for white middle-class men, and the variables were ill equipped to tap the life situation of African American men, although a number of studies that included blacks and whites had tested Type A or hostility and anger as related to blood pressure (for an excellent summary, see Kumanyika and Adams-Campbell 1991, 61–62).

In 1983, two conferences on CHD in black populations were held to address the unresolved and unknown issues related to CHD in blacks. As we can see from table 6.1, this was a time when the death rate from heart disease was becoming higher for black males than for white males. The conferences in 1983 mapped the scientific knowledge about the epidemiology of and risk factors for CHD among black populations and reviewed the validity of the available instruments and methodologies for future production of new scientific knowledge on CHD in black populations. The proceedings were assembled into a special issue of the *American Heart Journal* in 1984 (Johnson et al., 1984). In this issue Gillum and Liu reviewed the literature on CHD mortality among blacks between 1940 and 1978 and pointed to the widely held myth that blacks have lower rates of CHD than whites (1984, 728–729). The myth, they argued, has largely been a product of insufficient data, for three reasons: (1) studies before 1965 had been conducted in rural southern areas, (2) there was a lack of data on CHD incidence in blacks in northern urban areas in the 1960s and 1970s, and (3) inadequate access to medical care by blacks had probably resulted in underdiagnosis of CHD and in low recorded mortality and hospitalization rates. In 1985 and 1986 these themes were documented further and confirmed in two government reports on the health status of blacks and minorities (see Byrd and Clayton 2002, 370, 537).

In the same 1984 special issue of the *American Heart Journal*, Kasl summarized the latest knowledge about the impact of psychosocial factors on CHD in blacks: "Since the data on 'established' psychosocial risk factors are based on white populations, such evidence cannot hold firm promise that these are the relevant variables for blacks as well" (1984, 661). This view was echoed by James (1984b, 836), who referred to the report in 1981 of the Review Panel on Coronary-Prone Behavior and CHD, which had recommended that the Type A thesis be tested in blacks and other groups who differ from the middle- and upper middle-class white males studied up to that point (Review Panel on Coronary-Prone Behavior and Coronary Heart Disease 1981, 210). As James noted, no studies of the association between Type A behavior and CHD morbidity and mortality in blacks had been published by the early 1980s. For James, several methodological problems needed to be resolved in assessing Type A behavior in blacks. He suggested, "Thus, on logical grounds alone, the conceptual properties of type A behavior must be the same for blacks and whites, and initial efforts to identify the behavior pattern in U.S. blacks must proceed in a manner that is essentially faithful to the original conceptualization of Friedman and Rosenman" (James 1984b, 836).

In short, there was a need to conduct a study that would measure the personality risk factors for the development of heart disease among African American men. A term for the personality syndrome was soon found: *John Henryism*. The concept of John Henryism provided an acceptable answer about the coronary health of African Americans. It was a progressive model because, unlike the other constructs produced for white men, it recognized the economic location of African American men in the hierarchy of the labor market. Although not mentioned, institutional racism is a tacit theme in this model.

WHO IS THE MAN CHARACTERIZED BY JOHN HENRYISM?

The construct of John Henryism provided a conceptual scheme for interpreting the high rates of high blood pressure and hypertension among black men. The argument is based on the moral lesson of one of the legends of black oral history: an African American manual laborer, John Henry, races against a mechanical steam drill in his work, beats his enemy—the machine—and dies of overexertion. In the tale, John Henry emerges as an epic figure, refusing to bow to the power of organized society and the dehumanizing and deskilling effects of the reorganization of work. John Henry symbolizes the natural and moral hard man, who stands up against the displacement of black manual workers and farmers by machines and the market-oriented economic forces of white society (see Levine 1977, 420–429).

John Henryism is a synonym for active coping and was originally defined by its inventor as "an individual's self-perception that he can meet the demands of his environment through hard work and determination" (James et al., 1983, 263). A John Henry believes that he can control a hard situation through hard work and active striving. He does not, like Type C, fall into hopelessness, helplessness, and resignation. The construct valorizes a sense of "environmental mastery," especially the key issue of a "man's relationship to his work" (James et al., 1983, 274).

Later studies conducted by James and his colleagues have given slightly different definitions of John Henryism. One definition suggests that John Henryism "connoted a strong *personality* predisposition to cope actively with psychosocial stressors in one's environment" (italics added; James et al., 1987, 665). Another definition perceives John Henryism "as a strong *behavioral* predisposition to cope in an active, effortful manner with the psychosocial stressors of everyday life" (italics added; James et al., 1992, 59). There has been no scholarly debate whether the personality and behavioral components denote the same or different qualities. The same scale has been used in all the studies, with the result that the measurement device has tapped the same phenomenon, however the traits have been defined.

The John Henryism hypothesis predicts that a person who scores high in John Henryism (an active coping style of willingness to work hard and succeed), but has few resources (e.g., low education and low income) will be prone to health risks, operationalized as high blood pressure or hypertension.

In the original study John Henryism was measured by means of a Likert scale consisting of an instrument of eight items (James et al., 1983). When the sum of the items yields a high score, a high level of John Henryism is indicated. This high score is an indication of a man with "a strong sense of environmental mastery which is based, in part, on a single-minded determination to reach his goal" (James et al., 1983, 264). The first empirical study to test the John Henryism hypothesis was conducted with a sample ($n = 132$) of lower-income African American men in a poor semirural area of North Carolina in 1980 and 1981. The findings showed that men who had lower education levels, but scored high on John Henryism, had higher diastolic blood pressures than men who scored above the median on both measures.

In later studies the scale is called the John Henryism Scale for Active Coping, a twelve-item Likert scale, or the JHAC12. The scale emphasizes three themes: "efficacious mental and physical vigor; a commitment to hard work; and a single-minded determination to achieve one's goals" (James et al., 1987, 666). The responses range from "completely true" (score 5) to "completely false" (score 1), and the sum of the numerical values to the responses to the twelve items indicates the level of John Henryism. Affirmative answers mean a high score and high levels of John Henryism.

In the early 1980s when the John Henry measure was developed, the relationship between socioeconomic status and blood pressure and hypertension was typically an inverse one: blood pressure tended to be lower in higher socioeconomic groups than in lower socioeconomic groups. Nevertheless, blacks in all socioeconomic groups tended to have higher rates of hypertension than whites. The John Henryism thesis suggested that the expected inverse association would be stronger at higher levels of John Henryism than at lower ones. As the creators of the hypothesis phrase it, "The John Henryism hypothesis predicts that, in epidemiologic studies, the association between socioeconomic status and blood pressure will be modified by the individual's level of John Henryism" (James et al., 1987, 665).

When black subjects were grouped by degrees of John Henryism, socioeconomic differences in mean blood pressure only were shown among those who scored high in John Henryism (i.e., a commitment to a work ethic). Hypertension proved to be an even better marker: in the high-score John Henryism group, hypertension was nearly three times as prevalent as in the lower-socioeconomic-status group as in the higher-socioeconomic-status group (James et al., 1987). By contrast, in the low-score John Henryism group, there were no differences between the lower- and higher-socioeconomic-status groups in the prevalence of hypertension.

The John Henry man, then, is characterized by "hardness," which has been an icon of working-class culture. In his analysis of "hard men" and the embodiment of masculinity in American society, Jefferson shows that the hard man ethic has been a cultural revalorization of hardness as a consequence of industrialism and the power of the machine (1998). Hardness, he argues, has been emblematic of the brutal machine-driven reality for working-class men, rather than its antithesis. In this regard, hardness as a male characteristic has been an embodiment of the regulatory norm of working-class masculine behavior (see also Williams and Bendelow 1998, 126). In the words of Jefferson, hardness is "an interiorized quality extracted from risking the body in performance" (1998, 80–81). It is not merely the embodiment of physical force—a question of muscles—but also a kind of enduringness and mental toughness. It is in this latter meaning that the concept of hardness has merged with the construct of hardiness in the construction of the personality disposition known as John Henryism. Both concepts rest on a notion of men's perception of a moral self (e.g., Lamont 2000).

But John Henryism is also a cultural representation of black masculinity. John Henry is a social type who acts as a race man, that is, a racialized construction of a man (Drake and Cayton 1945, 394–395; Carby 1998). This construct is not gender neutral, but set in the order of race and gender in the United States. The John Henry is a type of black masculinity that embodies the ethical codes of white middle-class America. He stands for the "good" black man striving hard to achieve the values and goals of the white world, but denied full access and full agency as a man in the social and political order of dominant white masculinity. Translated into prosaic language, John Henryism is a personal predisposition to work hard despite the very low odds of ever achieving his goals.

Subsequent studies have failed to provide empirical support for the John Henryism hypothesis (e.g., Wiist and Flack 1992; James et al., 1992; McKetney and Ragland 1996). There are at least three reasons for the discrepant findings. One reason is socioeconomic. When the thesis was tested on a sample that included urban middle-class blacks, the relationship between mean blood pressure and John Henryism was not statistically significant.[2] Another reason is geographical. When urban and nonsouthern areas were included in later studies, the samples failed to provide evidence for the John Henryism hypothesis. A third reason is the age distribution of the samples. The hypothesis was not confirmed in a younger study population, a finding the researchers attribute to the low significance of both the independent and dependent variable. In a younger population, many had not yet finished their educations and attained their final occupational status. In addition, high blood pressure and hypertension have greater discriminatory power in an older than in a younger population (Wiist and Flack 1992; James et al., 1992; McKetney and Ragland 1996). Furthermore, a commitment to a work ethic, it has been suggested, is more characteristic of an older generation of people who have lived through harder times.

Gillum has suggested that the CHD rates of blacks have to be viewed in the light of social and demographic transitions in the black population since the early twentieth century (1996). He argues that the cohort effects have been more radical in the black population, which tends to be more heterogeneous, than in the white. Furthermore, regional differences are evident: Blacks born in the South have the highest mortality rates from CHD, those born in the Northeast have intermediate rates, and Caribbean-born and suburban middle-class U.S. blacks have the lowest rates (see also Corti et al., 1999, 311–312). Furthermore, studies have also pointed to the "mortality crossover" in CHD: older black men tend to have lower mortality than older white men (Corti et al., 1999, 308).

The results regarding the CHD rates for African Americans and whites and for different groups of blacks have provided further support for those who criticize the inclusion of race as a variable in epidemiological studies. The critics suggest that race has to be abandoned altogether in epidemiologic studies since it is not clear what it measures (Fullilove 1998; Stolley 1999). Others have been critical of those who suggest that race is subordinate to some more "real" and important social structure, such as social class. For example, the use of social class as a proxy for race has been criticized because the mere use of social class might tend to make the persistence of institutional racism invisible (e.g., Krieger 2000; Winant 2000). In this debate over the potential effects of using race in research, the American Sociological Association has encouraged collecting data and doing research on race because sociological scholarship on race provides scientific evidence in the debate over the social consequences of the existing categorization and perceptions of race (2003). The argument has been that "failure to gather data on this socially significant category would preserve the status quo and hamper progress toward understanding and addressing inequalities in primary social institutions" (2003). Further public support for research into the causes of racial inequalities in health is provided in the recently enacted Minority Health and Health Disparities Research and Education Act of 2000 (P.L. 106–525).

The use of different theories to explain the cardiovascular health of different social groups is further illuminated by research on Mexican Americans, a group constituting 11 percent of the American population (in 2001 there were, according to the U.S. Census, 37 million Latinos and 36 million blacks), but expected to constitute almost 25 percent by 2050. Compared to American white and black males, Hispanic males constitute a model of health. The death rate for diseases of the heart is considerably lower among Hispanic males than among white males and even lower than among white females (i.e., 213.8 per 100,000 resident population in 1998; see rates for whites in table 6.1).

Nevertheless, Mexican Americans are a heterogeneous group. As Jan Sundquist and Marilyn A. Winkleby's 1999 study shows, the CHD mortality risk is highest for U.S.-born Spanish-speaking men and women, intermediate for U.S.-born English-speakers, and lowest for Mexican-born Hispanics. The explanation given for the results has been a cultural one: the U.S.-born Spanish-speaking group is assumed to be culturally marginalized, whereas the healthiest, Mexican-born population, despite lower education levels, are assumed to derive their strength from their indigenous Mexican culture. This cultural explanation points to group-level cultural and social processes as explanatory factors for the

CHD rates among Mexican Americans. In sum, the Mexican culture, rather than any hypothetical ethnic personality type, has been presented as the reason for the CHD rates in research on CHD among Mexican Americans.

CONCLUSION

The high rates of CHD, especially of hypertension, among blacks have been a challenge to established medical knowledge that originally projected CHD as mainly a disease of white middle-class men. The construct of John Henryism provided a personality-focused model for interpreting and explaining the high rates of heart disease among African American men. The underlying idea of the John Henryism category was to construct an African American equivalent to Type A. In sociological terms, John Henryism is a race man, a type of embodied African American masculinity (Drake and Cayton 1945; Carby 1998), while Type A and the hardy man are embodiments of white middle-class masculinity. Both Type A and the hardy man are constructs developed in studies of white male executives, who furthermore were selected for the samples because they lived up to a traditional male breadwinner ideal. Type A man epitomizes the crisis of traditional masculinity, while the hardy executive emblematizes a well-adjusted conformer and the modern man as envisioned by Pleck (1976). The evaluation of the performance of these two types of men is based on how well they have managed to fit the contemporary white male sex role. The script of white masculinity rests on a notion of a certain autonomy and mastery of one's environment.

In the construction of John Henryism, the normative definition of (white) traditional masculinity was applied, even though the construct was developed for manual laborers. The John Henryism construct points to the possibility of multiple black masculinities, based on commitment to the work ethic and access to the means to achieve the culturally prescribed goal of individual success. Nevertheless, John Henryism is an idiom of the hard-working marginal black man. The normative discourse on masculinity as an active agent by definition pathologizes black males because the discourse is in conflict with the social position of most black men, who have little or no control over their social environment (Staples 1982, 2, and 1995a, 375).

The economic stratification of society by race and gender was considered, however, in the social construction of John Henryism, while the gender and racial hierarchies in society remained invisible in the construction of Type A and the hardy executive. The construction of both of the latter personality types rested on a fact taken for granted: at issue was a male who occupied a position of superordination in the gender and racial order.

John Henryism is a one-dimensional construct like hardiness: a man can record high or low scores on this one-dimensional scale. The scale measures a personality by degree rather than by different types—contrast this with, for example, Types A, B, and C. The high-score John Henry man is committed to hard work and to living up to the breadwinner ideal, like Type A man and the hardy executive. Both high-score John Henry men and Type A men are aggressive overachievers, characterized by overconformity with the ideals of white middle-class masculinity, which valorizes aggressive activity and mastery for the purpose of overcoming and controlling the environment. The "irrational" striving of both men is seen in medical terms as a health risk because they lack control over their life situations. The active coping style of the John Henry man is primarily a disease-promoting feature and not a health-promoting one like the active coping style of the (white) hardy man, as described in chapter 5.

There is a difference, however, in how much control the three types of men have over their lives. The lack of control displayed by Type A man is described as ontological: he seems to lack control over his inner self because he is other directed, rather than inner directed (e.g., Riesman 1950, 14–16). In their portrayal of Type A man, Friedman and Rosenman note the status anxiety of Type A man: "We have found after many years of studying the Type A man, that he either lost or never had any intrinsic 'yardstick' by which he can gauge his own fundamental worth to his own satisfaction" (1974, 75).

Type A man lacks what David Riesman called a "psychological gyroscope" (1950, 16). The inner-directed man obeys this internal piloting. Riesman suggests, "The inner-directed person becomes capable of maintaining a delicate balance between the demands upon him of his life goal and the buffetings of his external environment" (Riesman 1950, 16). Riesman here provides a working definition of the character of the hardy executive. An intrinsic motivation drives the actions of the hardy executive, who has thus constructed a sense of self-worth and self-control in his existence.

The hardy executive epitomizes white middle-class masculinity, a man who is not afraid of, but in fact feels challenged by, barriers to his operation and success in society. By contrast, the obstacles of the John Henry man, who is ambitious and is committed to the work ethic, are described in strictly instrumental and structural terms. The John Henry man is, like the hardy man, challenged by change and barriers to his success, but the John Henry is trapped by forces beyond his control. Unlike the opportunities awaiting the hardy executive if he works hard, the economic position and opportunities of the John Henry man are constrained by institutional racism. He is a marginal man in a society guided by an organization of super- and subordination of race and gender. Low-score John Henry men tend therefore to resort to a state of hopelessness and resignation, but high-score men feel challenged by the blockage of opportunities and tend to adopt a kind of aggressive striving that resembles Type A behavior (e.g., James et al., 1984; Jones 1993, 82). Later studies have explicitly looked at racism and discrimination as stressors for blacks (e.g., Harrell et al., 2003; Williams et al., 2003).

The John Henry man epitomizes the crisis of race and manhood for African American men and serves as yet another icon of the "perennial crisis of black masculinity" as perceived by the dominant society (e.g., Carby 1998, 6). By contrast, the hardy man, as chapter 5 shows, is the modern man who has re-captured his agency and a healthy male identity.

NOTES

1. The grassroots involvement introduced in the Community Health Planning and Services Act (P.L. 89–749) of 1965 was institutionalized in later federal health legislation, but a new terminology implicitly gave the lay involvement a new meaning. The lay representatives from the local area were now called "consumers," a term giving the impression that this was a group of middle-class people with purchasing power. For example, the HMO legislation (P.L. 93–222) of 1973 and the regional health planning agencies, the so-called Health Systems Agencies established as a result of the National and Health Planning and Resources Development Act (P.L. 93–641), of 1974 required a 51 percent representation of health care consumers on their boards.

2. The psychosocial stressors related to the social position of African American middle-class men have been supposed to cause health risks for them. More research on the coronary health of these men has been proposed (James et al. 1992 and James 1994).

Chapter Seven

The Construction of Categories and Measurements

Culture is like a map. Just as a map isn't the territory but an abstract representation of a particular area, so also a culture is an abstract description of trends toward uniformity in the words, deeds, and artifacts of a human group.

—Clyde Kluckhohn, *Mirror for Man*

THE SOCIAL CONSTRUCTION OF DIAGNOSTIC CATEGORIES

The scientific discovery of Type A was a mechanism through which emotional factors were given visibility as medical risk factors for developing CHD. Stress-related symptoms constituted an affliction that had not been visible to the eyes of the physicians before. The construction of Type A made transparent a certain type of male behavior and a certain type of masculinity that had not been conceptualized in medical terms. The medical argument was that Type A men were prone to develop CHD, a major killer of middle-aged men.

The argument presented throughout this volume is that medical knowledge and the vocabulary of psychology absorbed the features of major groups of men and integrated these representations into their scientific discourse. The variety of personality types in the gallery of human natures could therefore be interpreted in the words of Philip Rieff: "As cultures change, so do the modal types of personality that are their bearers" (1966, 2). What was new, however, was that these constructions of personalities were linked to the prospect of developing CHD at one point in the history of medical thinking in the United States.

The rise and fall of views in medical thinking is nothing new in the history of medicine (Cassell 1986). Still, in the area of CHD there has been a difference in the etiological discourse in the United States and in Europe, although they have something in common: CHD rates became a way of explaining and watching over an increase in men's deaths. But why was personality emphasized in the United States and not in Europe? Why is Type A not part of public discourse in Europe today as it is in the United States?

The medical thinking about CHD came to have a more individual focused and gendered impact in the United States than in most of Europe. In Europe the medical thinking captured a more collective notion. Sociologists who have looked at the history of CHD in the United Kingdom suggest that the rise of the "epidemic" of heart disease there was related to the medical discovery of heart disease in the 1940s. The impetus for this thinking was very much a product of a diffusion of post–World War II American influence in heart disease research in the United Kingdom. As Bartley shows, heart disease was seen as a disease of affluence and the price paid for rising standards of living, a way of life represented by the Americans (1985, 303–304). But the new categories also filled the doctors' and the population's need to find a cause for disease as biomedicine moved toward more disease-specific thinking. The new heart disease categories began increasingly to be used as cause-of-death definitions in death certificates. Myocardial infarction and CHD became new terms for explaining the "premature" deaths of British middle-aged men as life expectancy increased. Heart disease categories emerged, therefore, as reductionist categories for the cause of death in cases when an ambiguous heart-related problem was in question because the premature death of men was no longer accepted as merely part of the natural order.

The increasing rates of CHD in the United Kingdom have to a large extent been a social product, Bartley argues, and a way of organizing death (1985). The new diagnostic category of heart disease served the medical profession's need to find an appropriate label for deaths among a new generation of men who, after all, were living longer than previous generations of men had lived. This point is also made in Prior's study of death certificates in Belfast in the early 1980s (Prior 1985 and 1989). He shows that both cause of death and social class as shown in the statistics constitute reductionist categories that have served the need to find a simple classification within a complex social organization, the social function of which is to police and code deaths.

These British studies point to the social factors in the construction of mortality rates for men. These factors suggest that medicine is a broader social mechanism for watching over population groups, a trend that Armstrong has called "surveillance medicine" (1995). According to Armstrong, this trend means that medicine comes to exert tacit social control over the behavior of various groups, whose diseases and unhealthy behavior are put under medical surveillance. Armstrong suggests that "surveillance medicine" was an institutionalized part of the British national health system, a system that began to be established in 1912 through national health insurance and reconfirmed as a national health service in 1948 (1995). Public health and community health programs were part of how the welfare state ideology took shape in the health care arena.

In contrast to the collective orientation underlying welfare-state societies emerging after World War II in Europe (e.g., the United Kingdom, France, Germany, and the Scandinavian countries), medical practice in the United States remained private, and only limited public programs were initiated (e.g., Medicaid and Medicare, enacted in 1964, and some disease-focused programs like end-stage-renal-disease legislation, enacted in 1972).

In the United States, the individual-focused etiology of CHD has been grounded in the prevailing value structure in society and its health care system for a number of reasons. First, the personality-focused medical thinking had a cultural resonance in the United States with its tendency to valorize the achievement of individuals, instead of interpreting phenomena through the framework of social structures (a feature already pointed out by Parsons [1979]).

Even Friedman and Rosenman, in a popularized version of their thesis—a book entitled *Type A Behavior and Your Heart*—ask, "Why is Type A Behavior Pattern so exclusively a disease of our time?" (1974, 166). According to Friedman and Rosenman, "the most important reason, at least in the United States, is the transformation of nineteenth-century Yankee pragmatism into an unbridled drive to acquire more and more of the world's material benefits" (1974, 166). They continue, "When greed of this sort becomes indiscriminate, and cannot be sated by quality but only by numeration, the person involved has become a Type A" (Friedman and Rosenman 1974, 167). For Type A it is the material quantity, not the quality, of his achievements that matters, or as Friedman and Rosenman put it:

> The Type A man, after having striven for and obtained a certain *number* of dollars, doesn't care any more—and frequently even less—than the Type B about what use is made of the money. It is the *number* dollars, not the dollars themselves, that appease—but unfortunately only partially—the insecurity of the Type A man. (1974, 74)

Their analysis is that the behavior is part of the "historical national repertoire," as Michèle Lamont would say (1992).

Second, the etiological theory with a focus on personality and individuals also fitted the organizational structure of the medical and psychological profession in the United States, both of which operate from their private practice. Organized medicine has defended the entrepreneurial form of medical practice and argued that the "sacred trust" between the medical practitioner and his or her patient is the ethical foundation and guarantee of high-quality medical care (Harris 1969). An individual-focused epidemiological paradigm has therefore been congruent with a private practice system in which the individual patient consults with a private practitioner rather than visiting a local health center and its salaried medical staff, as in most European countries.

The emphasis on the private organization of health care was defended in the 1950s and in the early 1960s by the American Medical Association (AMA) as it tried to ward off a broader nationalized health insurance program or its more limited and targeted versions, Medicaid and Medicare. In the heyday of the Type A thesis, the principle of individualism and private medicine was touted in the inaugural address given by the president of the AMA and published in *JAMA*:

> If medicine is to serve the public in the future to the high degree that it has in the past, it must be united, standing strong and firm with a heart and conscience tuned to public need, with a respect for the rights and privileges of the individual, and with an abiding faith in our free competitive system of medical practice. (Welch 1964, 225)

Type A was the construct that helped private practitioners identify and diagnose a male patient afflicted with "hurry sickness" in their practice. The Structured Interview (SI) was the concomitant instrument that enabled the proper identification of Type A men. Soon other instruments to be used in typification emerged. The representatives of the etiological thinking linking a certain personality to CHD began to construct a variety of instruments to identify disease-prone or health-promoting psychological traits. The development of such instruments and new statistical techniques has produced and confirmed the proposed psychological categories.

The next section focuses on the key instruments and scales used in this kind of research and describes the constructive schemes for the production of the personality linked to CHD. A constructive scheme contains the practical rules for the production of data (Danziger 1990, 3). The following descriptions will provide information on how the personalities were constructed in the scientific discourse of medicine and health psychology. The concluding section of the chapter offers four different metaphors for how these measures assisted in the "discovery" of Type A man in medicine and his subsequent followers in health psychology.

HOW WERE THE MEASUREMENT INSTRUMENTS
FOR MAPPING TYPE A, HARDINESS, AND
JOHN HENRYISM DESIGNED?

The three psychological constructs analyzed in this book provide examples of the process that, according to the British sociologist Alan Petersen, has been largely hidden from the sociological eye (1998, 11). He laments that sociologists seldom illuminate what exactly is meant by the assertion that a body is socially constructed. In this book the social construction concerns the coronary-prone male body. The lack of descriptions of this process of social construction relates generally to the commonsense character of the phenomenon. As Berger and Luckman in their classic on the topic noted, a large part of the validity of knowledge of everyday life is taken for granted because it refers to the basic structures of everyday life (1967, 44–45). This has also been the case with the personality categories examined in this book. As Danziger suggests, a psychological theory operates on the basis of some preunderstanding of that which it is a theory of (1997, 6). This means that the categories are culturally valid because "what gives a particular sense to a term is the discourse of which it is a part" (Danziger 1997, 6). A psychological construct will therefore have a high validity because it is congruent with the cultural representation upon which it rests. About this epoch Danziger has noted, "In their pursuit of the project of personality measurement psychologists worked within a framework of assumptions that never had to be questioned because they were so widely held in the societies in which they operated" (1997, 128).

In the case of the social construction of the psychological constructs of Type A, hardiness, and John Henryism, the constructs rest on a popular discourse on masculinity. The cultural representations of masculinity became reified by incorporating them into scales and tests, and these measurement instruments reproduced the representations as psychological and medical facts. At the time of their construction, the personality types were seen as corresponding to the representation of their natural and generic kinds rather than located in a specific class, gender, and racial order. In scientific discourse, these cultural representations were further confirmed as natural categories—as part of nature—and outside of the structures of power organized around a hierarchical organization of class, race, and gender. The scales were designed to map a generic phenomenon, but the values of masculinity hidden in the constructs and the selection of white men only for the original samples made the instruments and the findings gendered and racialized.

Chapter 4 shows that Type A as a holistic concept was fragmented into numerous measurable components when the psychologists began to map and measure the Type A personality. Two approaches underlie this fragmentation. One is the perception of masculinity as a visible quality, or as Brittan has suggested, "Most discussions of masculinity tend to treat it as if it is measurable. Some men have more of it, others less" (1989, 1). Another is the risk-factor thinking about risks as measurable and preventable (see Aronowitz 1998).

In the original studies, the populations studied were middle-aged men. For example, a sample consisting of men only was used in the original SI developed by Friedman and Rosenman to identify Type A behavior. This was the case with the instrument to measure hardiness and the scale to measure John Henryism (see table 7.1; see also Kumanyika and Adams-Campbell 1991). Furthermore, the populations in the original studies were also socioeconomically and regionally biased. Friedman and Rosenman examined white male managers in California. The Framingham Heart Study, conducted in a suburb of Boston, included women, but hardly any African Americans. Hardiness was developed in a study of East Coast male executives working for Illinois Bell. The John Henryism scale was used for the first time in a sample of rural working-class African American men living in South Carolina.

Type A and Type B

The SI, designed for mapping Type A and Type B, contained a set of about twenty-five questions. The first questions relate to the respondent's type of work, and subsequent ones cover his sense of ambition, competitive nature, impatience, and time pressure. For example, the interviewer asks, "Do you think that you drive harder to accomplish things than most of your associates?" "When you play games with people your own age, do you play for the fun of it, or are you really in there to win?" "Do you eat rapidly? Do you walk rapidly? After you've finished eating, do you like to sit around the table and chat, or do you like to get up and get going?" "How do you feel about wait-

Table 7.1. Construction of Personalities: Key Measurement Instruments

Construct	Inventor	Instrument
Type A, B	Friedman and Rosenman (1959); Rosenman (1978)	Structured Interview
Type A	Jenkins (1966); Jenkins et al. (1979)	Jenkins Activity Survey
Type A	Bortner (1969)	Bortner Short Rating Scale
Type A	Haynes et al. (1978a; 1978b)	Framingham Type A Scale
Hardiness	Kobasa (1979); Kobasa et al. (1983)	12–18 standardized scales and tests
John Henryism	James et al. (1983; 1987)	John Henryism Scale for Active Coping

ing in lines: Bank lines, or Supermarket lines? Post office lines?" and "Do you have the feeling that time is passing too rapidly for you to accomplish all the things you'd like to get done in one day?" (Rosenman 1978, 68–69). The responses to these questions are recorded, but in addition, the interviewer uses a scoring sheet with a list of overt behavioral expressions and a scale of three to four adjectives describing the behavioral response.

The behavioral expressions listed on the standard scoring protocol are handshake, attitude, general appearance, motor pace, speech hurrying, voice quality, rhythmic movements (hands/feet), facial expression, laughter, fist clenching, sighing. For example, the handshake can be scored as "limp wrist, weak, average, strong" and the facial expression as "flat, expressive, lateral mouth, clenched jaw."

At the bottom of the sheet, the interviewer is asked to make a final impressionistic evaluation and define the person as A1, A2, X, or B (see Rosenman 1978, 67). The accuracy of the instrument is solid, according to Rosenman, who maintains that "it is generally possible to classify from 80% to 90% or more of subjects as predominantly Type A or Type B" (1978, 60).

In the late 1960s, the Bortner Short Rating Scale was developed. It uses fourteen items of a semantic-differential type (Bortner 1969). The respondent is asked to locate himself or herself in the space between two opposing extremes. This scale has not been used as much as the Jenkins Activity Survey scale, which became the standard Type A scale based on self-report.

C. David Jenkins of Boston University Medical School developed the Jenkins Activity Survey for Health Prediction, or the JAS test. The Jenkins Activity Survey was designed for adult working males and is a self-administered questionnaire of fifty-four items. For example, the respondent is asked, "Has your spouse or some friend ever told you that you eat too fast?" "How would your spouse (or best friend) rate your general level of activity?" (Responses include "too active," "too slow," "about average"). The more active style was indicative of a Type A behavioral pattern (Jenkins et al., 1979, see also Glass 1977, 27).

The applicability of the SI for groups other than male managers was challenged early and a shorter interview schedule—the Framingham Type A scale—was developed from the questionnaire administered to those who had been followed up on in the Framingham Heart Study. The purpose of the Framingham Type A scale is to measure Type A and B behavior. It consists of ten statements. The first part of the questionnaire comprises six areas concerning time pressure, competitive drive, and impatience. Five of these are "Having a strong need to excel," "Being bossy or dominating," "Usually feeling pressed for time," "Being hard driving and competitive," "Eating too quickly." The response choices range from "very well" (3) to "not at all" (0):

the respondent is asked to indicate "whether each trait describes you very well, fairly well, somewhat, or not at all." The sixth item is a question—"Do you get quite upset when you have to wait for anything?"—and is measured as yes (1) or no (0).

The second part consists of four statements eliciting reactions to work, with a separate addendum for housewives. The statements ask whether the respondent has at the end of the work day felt pressed for time, overexerted, bothered by work after work hours, or dissatisfied with work performance. The responses can be recorded as either yes (1) or no (0) (Weinrich et al., 1988, 178).

The responses to the ten statements are summed up. Type A people are defined as those whose scores are in the upper 50 percent of scores. The residual category with lower scores are then the Type B people (Weinrich et al., 1988, 166).

Hardiness

The measurement of the construct of hardiness has been complex since its inception. This personality style is, according to its originator, composed of three dimensions: control, commitment, and challenge. Each of these dimensions is measured by a pool of standardized tests that together compose an index proclaimed to be a measure of hardiness.

In the original study, Suzanne Kobasa used twelve standardized instruments (1979):

1. Four to test the control dimension (i.e., Internal-External Locus of Control Scale; Powerlessness Versus Personal Control Scale of the Alienation Test; the Achievement Scale and the Dominance Scale of the Personality Research Form; the Leadership Orientation Scale of the California Life Goals Evaluation Schedules)
2. Two to test the commitment dimension (i.e., the Alienation Test above and the Role Consistency Test)
3. Six to measure the orientation to challenge (i.e., Preference for Interesting Experiences Scale, Vegetativeness Versus Vigorousness Scale, Adventurousness Versus Responsibility Scale of the Alienation Test, Hahn's Scale of Security Orientation, Need for Cognitive Structure Scale, Need for Endurance Scale of the Personality Research Form).

The procedure was rather complicated. In the subsequent longitudinal study, Kobasa and her colleagues chose six scales: (1) the control dimension was measured by the External Locus of Control Scale and the Powerlessness Scale of the Alienation Test, (2) commitment was measured with the Alienation from Self and Alienation from Work scales of the Alienation Test; and (3) challenge was measured by the Security Scale and the Cognitive Structure Scale from the California Life Goals Evaluation Schedule and the Cognitive Structure Scale from the Personality Research Form (Maddi and Kobasa 1984, 97–98). The Cognitive Structure Scale was dropped later on, and the remaining five scales, comprising seventy-one items, became the Unabridged Hardiness Scale (UHS).

Each subscale is a negative indicator of hardiness, and the sum of the scales composes an index that is supposed to measure hardiness.

Funk (1992) has provided a comprehensive review of the development of the hardiness scale and its later descendants: the twenty-item Abridged Hardiness Scale (AHS), the thirty-six-item Revised Hardiness Scale (RHS), the fifty-item Personal Views Survey (PVS), and the forty-five-item Dispositional Resilience Scale (DRS). As Funk notes, the proliferation of scales makes the findings of hardiness research difficult to interpret because it is almost impossible to know whether the differences in outcomes are real or the artifact of the different scales used (1992, 336).

John Henryism

The first measurement device for mapping John Henryism was the John Henryism Scale with eight items (see James et al., 1983, 265). The scale consisted of eight statements to which the response options were "not true" (1), "somewhat true," (2) and "very true" (3). Total scores on this version of the John Henryism scale could range from a low of eight to a high of twenty-four. High scores indicated a strong sense of John Henryism.

In later studies the scale is called the John Henryism Scale for Active Coping, or the JHAC12, a twelve-item Likert scale, with responses ranging from "completely true" (5) to "completely false" (1) (see Weinrich et al., 1988, 177). The scale emphasizes three themes: hard work, goal orientation, and full agency (or, as the researchers grandly phrased the latter theme, "efficacious mental and physical vigor" [James et al., 1987, 666]). Attitudes toward hard work were measured, for example, by the following statements: "Hard work has really helped me to get ahead in life," "Very seldom have I been disappointed by the results of my hard work," and "When things don't go the way I want them to, that just makes me work even harder." Goal orientation was measured by, for example, this statement: "In the past, even when things got really tough, I never lost sight of my goals." Furthermore, the statements that capture men's sense of agency are worded as follows: "I've always felt that I could make of my life pretty much what I wanted to make of it," "I like doing things that other people thought could not be done," and "It's important for me to be able to do things the way I want to do them rather than the way other people want me to do them." The sum of the numerical response values indicates the level of John Henryism. Affirmative answers mean a high score and high levels of John Henryism. The maximum score is sixty and the minimum is twelve.

THE VALIDITY OF THE CONSTRUCTS

A number of studies have mapped the criterion-oriented validity of the scales measuring Type A, and most of them have concluded that the SI is the best measurement device (e.g., Edwards 1991). It has also been linked to CHD, in contrast to the tendency of the findings from the self-report measures to be null (Miller et al., 1991).

A study by Weinrich et al. was designed to test the validity and reliability of the Framingham Type A and John Henryism scales (1988). First, a factor analysis of the items in the two scales showed that the scales indeed measured different concepts. Second, race, gender, educational level, and working status were important variables for the John Henryism and Framingham Type A scales. For example, the features of strong John Henryism were more often found in males than in females, in blacks than in whites, and in the less educated than the more educated. When measured with the Framingham Type A scale, men were found more often to be Type A than were women, whites more often than blacks, and those with higher education more often than those with lower education. An interesting subgroup in the study was black men with high education. Like whites, these black men were not strong John Henryism types; instead, they were found to have the highest mean scores of all race and gender groups on the Framingham Type A scale, suggesting that they were very likely to be high-profile Type A men (Weinrich et al., 1988, 174).

The validity of the construct hardiness has been subject to serious criticism. This construct is operationalized by means of three separate concepts: control, commitment, and acceptance of change as a challenge. In the original study a total of twelve different standardized tests were used to measure the subcomponents of each of the three concepts (see Kobasa 1979, 5–6). An interesting methodological debate has been pursued over whether a single construct, hardiness, is indeed mapped by these three different characteristics (e.g., Hull et al., 1987; Funk 1992). Do the three characteristics have the same weight, or is one of them the crucial component? Furthermore, in the way that these three characteristics have been operationalized, most scales measure the negative dimension of the phenomenon, rather than the positive dimension upon which the whole concept is based. For example, it is assumed that a low score on the dimensions of powerlessness, alienation, and neuroticism are equivalent to a high propensity for the desired individual trait, hardiness (see Funk 1992). This is not necessarily the case, and the content validity of the measures is therefore questionable. In fact, criticism has also been directed at the use of different scales and tests in the various studies, a methodological problem that makes it difficult to compare the results of the studies on hardiness (Funk and Houston 1987; Funk 1992).

The measurement of personality dispositions in the Type A personality and hardy personality neglects the interference of certain values and attitudes. It is as likely that Type A men indulged in the unhealthy habits of the 1950s (smoking, fatty foods, little exercise) as it is that hardy men conformed to the value of physical fitness prevailing in the 1980s and 1990s. In that case, hardiness as a construct rests on another cultural tide—health as a value and individual asset among the middle class (Crawford 1980; Wagner 1997). The high CHD rates among middle-class men in the 1950s and the drop of the CHD rate among the same class of men two decades later could be interpreted in this light (see also Wiebe and McCallum 1986; Waldron 1995).

Furthermore, the John Henryism of African American men could also rest on other confounding variables (e.g., the attitudes of rural manual workers in the southeastern United States or a lack of access to health care, including preventive care). Furthermore the dependent variable, CHD, is related to the awareness among African American men of medical indications of the symptomatology of CHD. For example, a study of emergency room patients in Michigan (conducted in 1999) found that of those patients with the final diagnosis of myocardial infarction, 61 percent of African American patients attributed their symptoms to a gastrointestinal cause and 11 percent to a cardiac cause, while 26 percent of the white patients attributed their symptoms to a gastrointestinal cause and 33 percent correctly to a cardiac cause (Klinger et al., 2002). These figures suggest that African American patients are likely to get different treatments than whites because African Americans presenting with atypical symptoms may experience delays in getting a correct diagnosis and, hence, treatment for myocardial infarction.

CONCLUSION

At this point in our scientific journey of tracing the history of the Type A thesis and its operationalization by means of a number of scales and measurement devices, we can now facetiously, but still seriously, pose the question, Was there ever really a Type A man? In tracing the history of the rise of Type A man and his descendants, our accounts contain, in the words of a representative of science studies, Bruno Latour, four metaphors: the trail metaphor, the optical metaphor, the theater metaphor, and the industrial metaphor (Latour 1999, 140).

The trail metaphor is the way in which the two pioneering cardiologists themselves have interpreted their "discovery" of Type A man. Meyer Friedman and Ray Rosenman recall how the signs leading to the path of discovery were there, but they did not pay attention to them: "Like all our peers, we were not intellectually prepared twenty years ago to accept emotional stress as a relevant component for coronary heart disease" (1974, 55). Friedman and Rosenman's anecdote about the upholstery sign illustrates how they gradually became aware of the signs on the trail that led them toward their discovery:

> We had called in an upholsterer to fix the seats of the chairs in our reception room. After inspecting our chairs, he asked what sort of a practice we had. We said we were cardiologists and asked why he had wanted to know. "Well," he replied, "I was just wondering, because it's so peculiar that only the front edge of your seats are worn out." Had we been sufficiently alert, we might have thought about that chance remark and what it indicated about the behavior pattern of our coronary heart patients. (1974, 55)

They were then aided in following the right trail by the president of the San Francisco Junior League (a group of society women volunteers) and their husbands, whose dietary habits Friedman and Rosenman had studied. The results showed that there was no gender difference in fat intake and, thus, that men's proneness to heart disease could not stem from a higher intake of fat. The president of the league declared triumphantly that she had known this all along. She knew what was giving their husbands heart attacks: "It's stress, the stress they receive in their work, that's what's doing it." This comment was the crucial eye-opener for the researchers and led them to embark on the path of discovery. Friedman and Rosenman conclude, "And that's when our concept of Type A Behavior Pattern and its probable relationship to coronary heart disease was born" (1974, 56–57).

The trail metaphor considers the entity, Type A, to have existed as an independent object for the researchers to discover. In retrospect Friedman and Rosenman recall that the path to Type A behavioral pattern was there all along. The upholstery clue indicated that their male patients shared a certain behavioral pattern. It was their female informant who finally alerted them to men's stress at work, a comment that led them to a new theory of disease. The new medical theory, the stress theory of disease, framed their thinking, and they began to see the facts, the compulsive behaviors of male managers. The mapping of these habits enabled the researchers to gain access to Type A man. The SI was the pioneering instrument that made possible the access to the different behavioral patterns, Types A and B. The Jenkins Activity Survey, the

Bortner scale, and the Framingham Type A scale enabled further precision in the identification of these two types.

The optical metaphor is another way of describing the invention of Type A man and subsequent types of personalities. According to this metaphor, there were fragments of behaviors, but a certain gaze and way of seeing made Type A man as an entity visible. The medical and psychological gaze upon a certain type of men—white-collar men—constructed Type A man and Type A personality in medical and psychological discourse, respectively. Chapter 3 presents a Foucauldian interpretation: the phenomenon is seen as constructed in discourse, and the medical gaze unveiled Type A. The scales and measurement instruments, described in this chapter, constituted the discursive technique—the optical instrument—that made Type A and other personality types visible to other researchers as well and enabled a testing of the personality thesis to begin.

The theater metaphor, or metaphor of staging, is used by Latour to privilege the role of the researcher as a stage manager in the presentation of the research findings. Some facts are presented in the spotlight on the stage; others are kept backstage. I use the metaphor slightly differently. I apply the theater metaphor to the way that social scientists have constructed the social dimension of male behavior defined as Type A. The theater metaphor does not address the biological dimension of Type A, but tries to explain how and why social definitions of gender are embedded in seemingly biological sex categories. The theater metaphor is represented by those social scientists who see masculine behavior as either a script or a performance. Sex-role theory has presented male behavior as a script, a male sex role, that is learned and followed by men. The performative notion is represented by those social scientists who present gender as a social construct. According to this notion, gender is not merely a representation but also a social process of performing gender at different levels of society (Lorber 1993 and 1994; Kimmel 2000). Gender in this way becomes a key organizing principle in social and economic life. By making the values and belief systems visible in how Type A has been operationalized in scientific research, the researcher points to the way that social definitions are embedded in categories of medical knowledge. The discovery or invention of Type A was therefore related to the social definition of masculinity at the time, a definition and representation of racialized, classed, and gendered individuals that came to be integrated into medical knowledge.

The industrial metaphor treats men's bodies as the raw material from which a discursively constructed body appears. Type A man is a discursively inscribed male body. The paradox is that the transformation of this male body in scientific discourse turns this body, Type A man, into a more real phenomenon than it was before. This is the argument presented by Danziger (1997), Aronowitz (1998), and Rose (1997), when they point to the historicity of categories. This notion has two implications.

First, they argue that medical and psychological categories are historically constructed objects in the scientific enterprise of medicine and psychology. This chapter has reviewed the constructs and the instruments that have operationalized the personality types. The review shows how the instruments develop from being rough measurement devices, like the SI, to becoming evermore complex summations of a number of standardized psychological scales, exemplified in the measurement of hardiness.

Second, although the psychological categories are discursive categories and representational, they become constitutional. The discursive male, Type A, materializes through an embodied and gendered Type A man. As Rose suggests, psychological categories have been the necessary "grammar" through which a modern self has been both constructed and embodied (1997). In a similar way, the attributes of Type A, as described and confirmed by the psychological scales, became how people constructed and experienced themselves as the entity labeled Type A.

Throughout my account of the scientific enterprise of the rise and fall of Type A and of the emergence of new constructs to confirm the old hypothesis, I have argued that gender, class, and race are embedded in the personality constructs and their operationalization in scientific research. The constructs reflect normative notions of prevailing racial and gender categories and hierarchies. In this regard the use of the personality constructs in scientific research has not only produced scientific "facts," but also reflected and confirmed the social consequences of existing categorizations and perceptions of race and gender.

Here we are reminded by Danziger's claim (1997, 192) that the only reality that the psychological categories reflect is a cultural reality. Using this way of thinking, I have argued that Type A was not an independent natural object out there to be discovered. Instead, medicine transformed a culturally grounded representation of masculinity into a medical category called Type A. The scales and measurements have confirmed the gendered, classed, and racialized categories that existed as prescientific categories in public discourse. The links between scientific discourse and public discourse have been multidirectional: sociocultural contexts have influenced scientific knowledge production, and scientific discourses have constructed social reality (see Shim 2002, 144).

Whichever of the four metaphors above one adopts, one has to recognize that the personality categories examined in this volume are seemingly unmarked and disembodied. The science of the enterprise has made the aspect of gender, class, and race invisible, because the task of the scientific endeavor was to map or unveil a generic category. The transformation of the embodied and marked character of men to generic kinds has been through a psychologistic framework. Psychologism is a framework that has reduced the structural aspects of the categories to psychological and innate traits of individuals. The unmarkedness of the personalities by gender and race has been a way of maintaining men's location in the prevailing gender, racial, and economic order (see Butler 1993; Hearn 1996; Robinson 2000; Davis 2002). The unmarkedness renders invisible social relations of power. This view of the science of Type A and its descendants can be called the naturalization metaphor.

In the next chapter we turn to the question of the structural characteristics of the social types of men who have been portrayed as a Type A man, a hardy executive, and a John Henry.

Chapter Eight

Types of Masculinities:
Class, Race, and Men's Health

The white-collar people slipped quietly into modern society. Whatever history they have had is a history without events; whatever common interests they have do not lead to unity; whatever future they will have will not be of their own making.

—C. Wright Mills, *White Collar: The American Middle Classes*

PSYCHOLOGICAL CATEGORIES AS SOCIAL CATEGORIES

While sociologists have pointed to the social construction of medical and diagnostic categories, this work has often been done on an abstract level. Type A personality, the hardy personality, and John Henryism provide concrete, but individualized, explanations of social differences in health. In personality-focused etiological models, personality is viewed as an innate and individually based risk factor for CHD. In such models the social differences in cardiovascular disease rates among men have tended therefore to be explained by differences in individual personality dispositions. Yet, the structural locations of the types of men, briefly referred to in the foregoing chapters, pose for them certain strains and dilemmas caused by their social positions in the institutional framework of society. The purpose of this chapter is to deconstruct the three major personality types and make transparent the maleness of these constructions, but also to locate them as social categories of men in the economic and social order.

The relationship between structure and culture and its influence on social action is a classic theme in sociology. Parsons's oversocialized and conformist individual became the target of criticism, and new approaches were introduced in

the 1950s. Merton's goals-and-means scheme was a way of addressing the issue of social change, while still using a structural functionalist approach (1957).
According to Robert Merton, there are culturally prescribed goals and socially
structured channels for realizing these aspirations, but there is also differential
access to the legitimate means for achieving these goals. Merton set out to explore modes of adaptation to contradictions in cultural and social structures
(1957, 140). He offered a typology of various types of adaptations to contradictions between the cultural and social structures. He focused on types of individual adaptations constructed as role behaviors because, as Merton states,
"we are not focusing on character or personality types" (1957, 152). The social
types Merton constructed never seem to have found their way into medicine
(1957, 140), but the personality types used in medical discourse for predicting
men's coronary-prone health can easily be mapped using his taxonomy.

The Mertonian goals-means scheme will be used here for heuristic purposes: to illustrate the theoretical assumptions of sex-role theory embedded
in the personality types constructed in medical and psychological discourse.
As table 8.1 shows, this goals-means scheme serves as the underlying eval-
uative tool of the social behavior of the different personality types. The fit
between the personality types and Merton's scheme suggests that sex-role
theory, especially the assumption about the instrumental character of men's
role, is the theoretical and explanatory framework that underlies the personality constructs.

According to Merton, culturally prescribed aspirations in the United States
are shaped by "success values" (1957, 170). There are legitimate means of
achieving the cultural goals, and goal-striving is behavior based on rational
calculation. As table 8.1 shows, Type B and the hardy man are rational and
conformist actors. Both men are committed to the culturally prescribed goal
of success, and they use legitimate means to achieve these goals. The hardy
man captures the spirit of rationalism and innovation, which seems to be a
quality missing among Type A men. While the hardy man embraces the entrepreneurial spirit, he also seems to carry the social virtues of a sense of duty
to others, reliability, and cooperativeness, qualities that the self-possessed and
antisocial Type A man lacks.

**Table 8.1.   A Typology of Masculine Coronary-Prone Personalities in Medical and
Psychological Discourse as Related to Merton's Scheme**

Personality	Cultural Goals	Institutionalized Means	Social Behavior
Type B, hardy men	+	+	Conformism
Type A	−	+	Social ritualism
John Henryism	+	−	Overconformity
Type C	−	−	Retreatism

Type A man is committed to success values, but he does not act rationally. He is too focused on the means of hard work, and his aggressive, competitive behavior makes him lose sight of the goal towards which he is striving. His frenzied striving becomes irrational and takes its toll on his health. Similarly, the John Henry man is committed to the extrinsic rewards of success. He works hard to achieve them, but he lacks the normal means, such as education and income, to achieve the aspired-to cultural goals. The fact that he restricts his action to the legitimate means makes him prone to hypertension or high blood pressure.

For Type C man, the cultural goals and institutionalized means are far from a reachable reality, and he is characterized by helplessness and hopelessness and tends to retreat into a state of resignation—retreatism.

The strength of Merton's scheme is that it offers a taxonomy of values and social types. But as chapter 2 suggests, the weakness of sex-role theory is that it makes invisible the character of the economic, gender, and race order. The next section identifies and locates the personality types in a certain institutional order.

THE TYPIFICATION OF MEN AND THE RELATED INSTITUTIONAL CONTEXT

The relationship between the self and social order is a classic theme in the social-interactionist literature. The founding concepts of the discipline were presented by Charles H. Cooley in *Human Nature and the Social Order,* which appeared in 1902. In chapter 9 of that book, Cooley, under the heading "Leadership and Personal Ascendancy," explores the relationship between personality and social change. He argues that the self is never an isolated abstraction, even if a person is a leader, but relates to the needs of a particular social structure. For Cooley the "leader is a cause, but, like all causes we know of, he is also an effect" (1902, 357). Cooley notes:

> Every leader must also be a follower, in the sense that he shares the general current of life. He leads by appealing to our own tendency, not by imposing something external upon us. Great men are therefore the symbols or expressions, in a sense, of the social conditions under which they work, and if these conditions were not favorable the career of the great man would be impossible. (1902, 354)

The theme of the self and social structure, in particular as related to work and organizations, became a central theme in modern sociology. The later Chicago school of sociology, represented by Everett Hughes (1945) and his disciple C. Wright Mills (1951; Gerth and Mills 1954), reflected on the char-

acter of self and the status and dilemmas of people working in the modern organization of work (at the time, the sort of organization of work that produced
the Type A kind of men). For Hughes, the structure of work provides a set of
positions with their demands and expectations—a master status—into which
the individual has to fit (1945). The master status was not only gendered, but
also related to a position in the class and racial order for which white middle-
class men were fit.

When five years later Mills turned his sociological gaze on white-collar
men, he saw that the new demands of the changed economy confronted white
middle-class men (a segment he called the new "Little Man") with institutional dilemmas. In *White Collar: The American Middle Classes*, Mills examines in a Weberian way the characters of various strata in American society and their attitudes and social behavior (1951). In his later work, *Character
and Social Structure: The Psychology of Social Institutions*, Mills adopts, together with Hans Gerth, a social psychological approach to character (1954).
As Mills suggested, the task of sociology should be to "trace the shiftings of
psychic strains and stresses which are deposited in various groups within society by the structural changes which it undergoes" (Gerth and Mills 1954,
15). A sociological understanding of human conduct implies an effort to "'locate' the human being and his conduct in various institutions, never isolating
the individual or the workings of his mind from his social and historical setting" (Gerth and Mills 1954, 3). In my analysis of the psychological constructs that depict men's personality, I am using Mills's concept of institutional order (see table 8.2), defined as "all those institutions within a social
structure which have similar consequences and ends or which serve similar
objective functions" (Gerth and Mills 1954, 25).

Almost fifty years later, Richard Sennett continues this tradition and examines the sociohistorical changes of capitalism and the psychological
processes that form the characters of individuals and their attitudes to work

**Table 8.2.   The Institutional Context of the Type A Man, the Hardy Executive, and
John Henry Man**

Institutional Order	Type A Man	Hardy Executive	John Henry Man
Economic order	Entrepreneurial and corporate capitalism	Post-Fordist market capitalism	Dual-labor capitalism
Social order	—	—	—
Racial order	White men	White men	African American men
Class order	Middle class, white collar	Middle class, white collar	Working class, blue collar
Gender order	Traditional man	Modern man	Traditional man

and self (1998). C. Wright Mills had pointed to the bewilderment of modern white-collar men as they were trying to set out their life narrative and make it into a coherent and meaningful life story, as the quotation in the beginning of this chapter suggests. Sennett's tone is even more pessimistic (1998). He identifies late-twentieth-century capitalism as a capitalism characterized by flexibility and the uncertainty of short-term jobs. This economic condition, Sennett argues, provides workers, like the Millsian Little Man, with no opportunities to set out a life narrative that will progress in a linear, career-like fashion. Above the Little Man is, in the words of Sennett, the "Davos man" of today's global capitalist enterprises that set the structural conditions of the economic order (1998, 61). The Davos man is a reference to the world's corporate leaders who together with world government leaders gather annually for a weeklong conference called the World Economic Forum, held at a ski resort in Davos, Switzerland. According to Sennett, the Davos moguls constitute "a kingdom of achievers, and many of their achievements they owe to the practice of flexibility" (1998, 61).

As Sennett sees it, the social structure of current short-term-job capitalism has corroded the moral character of small entrepreneurs, whom Max Weber had portrayed as the primary carriers of the spirit of capitalism. As Sennett phrases it, "How can long-term purposes be pursued in a short-term society? How can a human being develop a narrative of identity and life history in a society composed of episodes and fragments?" (1998, 26).

If one deconstructs the psychological categories—the Type A man, the hardy executive, and the John Henry man—and defines them in light of their contemporary master status, these men can be positioned in the institutional order of a specific social and historical setting. They match the social categories of men located in certain positions in two institutional orders: the economic and the social order.

Table 8.2 shows the location of the Type A man, the hardy executive, and the John Henry man in two different institutional orders—the economic and social order. These men's struggle for control over external goals gets translated into an internal struggle over their tormented selves, carefully measured as the behavioral and attitudinal expressions of individual men in the medical and psychological discourses on the personality predispositions for CHD.

The institutional changes and concomitant dilemmas for the men who occupied the positions of privilege in the 1950s were not explicated in the medical discourse on Type A. Type A man is experiencing the strain between the traditional and modern male sex role. He has been socialized according to the values of traditional masculinity, and his behavior and values reflect his adherence to this role. Nevertheless, the values and the economy are paving the way for a new economic actor: the modern man. Type A man's sense of a lack of control seems to have coincided with the fall of the last remnants of old-time, cottage-industry, entrepreneurial capitalism in the American economy. Type A man had survived the Great Depression, an era from which he carried the cultural baggage of a tarnished masculinity. For white men, the Great Depression had challenged the normative task to live up to the breadwinner role, regardless of their work ethic. Although World War II resurrected and again legitimized traditional masculine values, the postwar years and the 1950s changed the economy, and a crisis of traditional masculinity was impending (Pleck 1981, 159; Kimmel 1997). The 1950s were also the years of McCarthyism, which further added to the pressure to conform to traditional ideals, including the nuclear family and traditional sex roles.

In the early 1980s, the hardy man enters the psychological discourse. He displays the sex-role attributes of the modern man as envisioned by Pleck (1976). The hardy man works in a post-Fordist economy, characterized by job insecurity and flexibility. Nevertheless, the hardy man does not perceive this economy as a threat, but rather as a challenge. He has the adaptive coping and interpersonal skills needed in the post-Fordist economy. He is also an icon of the new ethical regime of work ethic and self-regulation that serves as the underlying moral foundation of the neoliberal approach to the economy and government (Rose 1999; Lemke 2001). In the American version of the neoliberal approach, the market serves as the organizing principle for the society, and the social sphere is redefined as a form of the economic domain. Self-discipline and free, rational, and responsible actors constitute the governing regime of the neoliberal society. As Thomas Lemke observes, "The key feature of the neo-liberal rationality is the congruence it endeavours to achieve between a responsible and moral individual and an economic-rational actor" (2001, 201). In this regard, the hardy man encapsulates the competence of the rational and responsible individual, a kind of ethical regime that shifts the regulation of the state to the self-regulation of individuals through their enactment of the ethic of entrepreneurship. Within this ethical regime, hardiness is a representation of self-discipline—a kind of self-control that Max Weber defined as the Protestant ethic (1958) and that Foucault called the technology of the self (1988). Not only does the valorization of hardiness promise the prevention of CHD among the key economic actors—the hardy executives—but self-discipline promises the health of society as well.

In addition to hardiness, the construct of John Henryism appeared in the early 1980s. The John Henry man is an African American who works on the periphery of a dual-labor market economy and is doomed to a dead-end or short-term job, if he ever has a job.

Table 8.3 lists the behavioral and emotional reactions to the institutional dilemmas of the social category of men portrayed here as the Type A man, the

Table 8.3. The Behavioral and Attitudinal Characteristics of the Type A Man, the Hardy Executive, and the John Henry Man

Expressions	Type A Man	Hardy Executive	John Henry Man
Motivation	Extrinsic	Intrinsic	Extrinsic
Morality	Hostile, selfish	Responsible, committed	Moral, "hard" man
Goals and orientation	Success, anxiety	Success, challenge	Success, ambition
Behavior	Social ritualist	Conformist	Overconformist
Attitude to change	Feeling threatened	Adaptive coping, problem solving	Adaptive coping, but feeling trapped by forces beyond own control
Autonomy	Lacking control	In control	Lacking control
Agency	Crippled	Full	Blocked
Health behavior promoting	Disease-disposition stress	Health-promoting	Disease-promoting stress

hardy executive, and the John Henry man. In psychological discourse the emotional reactions were framed as a personality, but a sociological reading of the emotions and the behavior of these men show them as embodied selves with different capacities for social agency. The high-score John Henry man is committed to hard work and to the breadwinner ideal, like Type A man. Both high-score John Henry men and Type A men are plagued by overconformity to the ideals of American white masculinity. Both Type A and John Henry men are driven by a so-called maximax strategy, which means that they strive for maximum rewards at maximum expense (Young 1980, 139).

Both John Henry and Type A men have little control over their life situations, and their "irrational" striving is seen as a medical risk. There is a difference, however, in the extent of the control that the two have over their lives. Type A man's lack of control is existential: he seems to lack control over his inner self, while he has achieved and continues to strive for external goals. By contrast, the John Henry man's obstacles are strictly instrumental and structural: he has a low education or low income level, or both, which prevents him from being able to achieve external success goals. The John Henry man has little control over his external environment.

Each of the three types of men—Type A man, the hardy man, and the John Henry man—is committed to success, and the constructs emphasize drive and goal attainment as the major values of these men. The hardy executive is a construct that connotes the victorious man who has overcome the masculine insecurity plaguing the Type A man. The hardy man sets his own pace, and he is characterized by self-control and self-regulation. He has the kind of character—hardiness—that Sennett thought had withered away with the new short-term-job capitalism (1998). While both Type A man and the hardy man struggle with the traditional notions of autonomy and self-control as part of the essence of manhood, the John Henry man is also guided by these values, but his lack of success is explained in structural terms. His location in the job market is characterized by racial discrimination, a structural feature he is not willing or able to identify. Instead, he is trapped in a male mystique and takes his lack of success to be a product of his personal failure as a man.

The three psychological categories—Type A, hardiness, John Henryism— offer a psychological theory of men's health. Through the lens of a psychological discourse, men are constructed as victims of a working life that is interpreted as curtailing their agency. The prerequisite for men's health is a situation where a man as an active self has the kind of autonomy and mastery over his external conditions that enables him to feel in control of his life. But who is this mythic man? Is he the bearer of the idea of a presocial, archaic human nature? This mythology is based on an essentialist view that men's full agency, in the form of "purposeful outward intentionality" (Whitehead 2002, 200), constitutes the essential core of their identity as men. This mythology is also the content of a "doctrine of self-control" that has served as the normative guideline for most American men (Kimmel 1997, 45), a mythology that has had a powerful appeal in constructing the identity of the "normal" American male.

The blocked agency of the John Henry man and the Type C man leads to their experience of low esteem as men. By contrast, the hardy man seems to capture the characteristics of full agency, in contrast to Type A. The construct of hardiness has restored the masculine subject by promoting a type of male who has recaptured his full agency. The hardy man is a hard-working man who has adopted a rational and problem-solving approach to changes at work. He is a carrier of the kind of innovative spirit associated with the classic spirit of capitalism. These qualities make him able to cope with the kind of flexibility that characterizes the labor processes, labor markets, and labor in a post-Fordist economy (see Harvey 1989; Sennett 1998). The hardy man also professes the kind of special virtues that writers with libertarian views, like Francis Fukuyama (1995, 46), claim are essential qualities of economic actors in an economy having, in this way, a built-in potential to prosper. According to Fukuyama, in a growth economy the major economic actors should not only be committed to a work ethic but, more importantly, they should profess certain social virtues, like honesty, reliability, a sense of duty to others, and cooperativeness. Such virtues constitute the necessary cultural component of trust and social capital that, Fukuyama argues, are needed for a network structure of capitalism to emerge, be sustained, and prosper. As Fukuyama puts it, "A healthy capitalist economy is one in which there will be sufficient social capital in the underlying society to permit business, corporations, networks, and the like to be self-organizing" (1995, 356).

Back in the 1950s, when the new economic order of corporate capitalism was making the small entrepreneur obsolete and the new order of post-Fordism was on the brink of developing, there was no place for Type A men. In such an economy Type A man, encapsulating traditional masculinity, was an anachronism. Type A man was obsessed with hard work, but he had lost the problem-solving skills and creative imagination that constituted the hallmark of the classic spirit of capitalism. His antisocial and self-possessed attitudes made Type A man ill equipped for a modern economy based on flexibility and teamwork. The new economic order fostered a new type of manager and worker, a modern man described by the economic observers referred to above—descriptions that range from the neo-Marxist interpretations offered by David Harvey and Richard Sennett to the neoliberal communitarian outlook represented by Francis Fukuyama.

One does not have to be a Marxist to see the historic dynamics of economic relations and to identify the forces of social structure rather than the psychological essence of an economic actor as the mover of society. In this regard, the Marxist notion of alienation is a useful construct and in need of resurrection: despite its underlying essentialist notion of the existence of a presocial, pure inner self untarnished by the forces of capitalism, the concept of alienation addresses the ontological problems of the victimized self within the framework of work and economic change. The concept combines the levels of agency and structure by locating the sense of identity and consciousness in material conditions that are shared by individuals who in this way constitute a group that in itself has a potential to act as a group for itself.

The personality-focused theories of CHD fixed the gaze on the inner life of the self, men's interior and emotional self, rather than raising the issue of the wounded self as a structural problem. The psychologism and methodological individualism made the institutional order and the historic setting of these men invisible (see table 8.1). In the American medical discourse on Type A, the coronary health problem of white middle-class men was interpreted as being located in their personality. The psychologization of the health problems of American middle-class men turned masculinity to a personal health hazard and a health cost. Type A man was constructed as a visibly wounded form of white masculinity, while the hardy man has added legitimacy to the core values and meanings of dominant masculinity in American society. This psychological construct has demedicalized masculinity: hardiness has restored and revitalized the values of maleness—ambitions, self-reliance, autonomous responsibility—in the name of health. The modern man has learned through the concept of hardiness about the key features of a healthy male identity for the post-Fordist era.

CONCLUSION

This chapter locates the social categories of men introduced in the CHD literature—the Type A man, the hardy executive, the John Henry man—in the prevailing economic and social order. As the foregoing chapters show, different frameworks have been used in the medical discourses on CHD. Chapter 6 shows that only one of the frameworks—the personality of John Henryism applied to explain the cardiovascular risk factors among African American men—has indicated the existence of the larger institutional frameworks of gender, class, and race, while the CHD rates among Mexican American men have mainly been interpreted in terms of intergroup relations and cultural factors. Chapters 3, 4, and 5 show that white (middle-class) men's health has not explicitly been located in any of the foregoing three institutional frameworks, but has been seen as related to innate personality traits.

This chapter illustrates how sex-role theory and the notions of men's instrumental tasks, exemplified in the Mertonian goals-means scheme, underlie the personality theories. Chapter 2 shows that liberal critics of the traditional male sex role in the 1970s saw the male attributes of hostility and competitive drive as merely values and attitudes that could be unlearned and another less aggressive male role adopted (see Messner 1998). The hardy executive is emblematic of the notion that men can be socialized or resocialized to new behaviors and attitudes, while leaving the underlying gender order intact and unchallenged. The contemporary middle-class man—the hardy executive— can now be committed to the work ethic without health consequences, because he has a "hardy personality style" that "function[s] as a resistance source in the encounter with stressful events" (Kobasa et al., 1982, 169). He has control over his external and internal self and presents himself as emotionally balanced and equipped with the necessary social skills required in today's working life.

Chapter Nine

Conclusion

Few of [the things we all find stressful] are "real" in the sense that that ze-
bra or that lion would understand. In our privileged lives, we are uniquely
smart to have invented these stressors and uniquely foolish enough to have
let them, too often, dominate our lives. Surely we have the potential wisdom to banish their stressful hold.

—Robert Sapolsky, *Why Zebras Don't Get Ulcers: A Guide to Stress,
Stress-Related Diseases and Coping*

MEN AS THE VICTIMS OF HEART DISEASE

Fifty years ago heart disease was seen as reaching epidemic proportions. Infectious diseases, especially tuberculosis, were no longer the major killers.
People began to live longer and became sufferers of chronic illness. The rise
of chronic diseases, like CHD, was a product of this epidemiological and demographic transition. But CHD was a major killer of *men,* and the question
was, Why were *they* the victim of this disease? Perhaps even more importantly at issue was the question, Why are hard-working, middle-class, middle-
aged men dying of heart disease? From a sociological point of view, the disease was hitting the core of what has been called "hegemonic masculinity"
(Connell 1987). The rising prevalence and death rates of CHD exposed the
vulnerability of these men, and the disease was thus a threat to the social order of the dominant groups of men.

The early etiological thinking on heart disease focused on men as consumers: the reason for men's proneness to CHD was that they were consuming too much fat and sugar, and they smoked. This consumption pattern among
men was perceived as the major risk factor for developing heart disease. Yet

some research failed to prove a direct connection between these factors and the onset of heart disease. A new medical thinking emerged, and it placed men in the sphere of production: men's health problems were related to work. It was the emotional component of modern work that made its major actors, male executives, ill. Furthermore, it was the personalities drawn to the material success promised by this mode of economic production who were the victims of this very economy. It was these men who became the victims of heart disease.

This book has looked at the history of the "heart failure epidemic" in the United States since the 1950s onward, especially at the notions of men as the primary victims of this disease. I have traced the genesis of CHD and how the cause of this disease has been constructed in medical discourse. I have focused on the early etiological theories that tried to grapple with the reasons for the rapid rise of CHD among men, especially white middle-class men. In the 1950s, a new theory suggested that a certain type of behavior among these men predicted the incidence of heart disease. A new risk factor, Type A, emerged in medical discourse, and the Type A personality was later constructed in psychological discourse.

This book is based on two approaches. The first approach is methodological. The method used in this book is a meta-analysis of scientific texts in medical and psychological discourse. The purpose has been to unravel the historical epistemology of personality as a construct in American medicine and the use of this construct as a medical risk factor for men's propensity to get CHD. The analysis presented has pointed to the need to see medical categories in a historical perspective and as socially constructed categories. The book has focused on the "domain of constructions" (Danziger 1990, 2) of a certain set of personalities thought to be related to the onset of CHD.

The second approach is the deconstruction of the notion of men as victims. The victimization view has interpreted men's wounded self as symptomatic of men's lack of agency as autonomous social actors. Normative masculinity states that a man should have control of his inner self and of his external environment. Lack of self-control has been interpreted as an indication of an emotionally wounded and pathologized man. These notions have been expressed in a medicalization of middle-class men's agency.

The underlying explanatory framework for understanding and explaining men's health in the past has been sex-role theory. While feminist theorizing on women's health has pointed to this thematic theoretical stream in most research on women's health (e.g., Lorber and Moore 2002; Annandale and Hunt 2000), the allegedly gender-neutral research on men's health, particularly research on CHD, has also been framed within the tradition of sex-role theory. In fact, research on men's coronary health in the 1950s and 1960s preceded research that identified the female embeddedness of the sick role.

MEN'S HEALTH AS AN UNDERRESEARCHED ISSUE

Men have been the model of health in medicine. This was the picture promoted by women's health advocates in the 1970s. It was argued that men's bodies have constituted the generic standard of health in medical texts and medical knowledge. The major argument of this book is that the medical knowledge of men's health was also biased and that men's health problems were also medicalized, but in a different way than women's. While women's reproductive health matters were the predominant object of medicalization, for men it was the behaviors and attitudes related to CHD that became the target of medicalization. As I have shown, Type A represented a certain type of masculine behavior that was connected to white men, specifically white-collar men. The foregoing chapters have illustrated how the gendered and racialized issue hidden in the studied entities were psychologized and naturalized as part of the scientific enterprise.

A number of issues have surfaced in the discussion in the foregoing chapters, but have not been addressed explicitly. I will address three of those issues in this concluding chapter.

The first issue: In my analysis of the Type A thesis in the foregoing chapters I have at several points suggested a link between the economic order and the social order and between these orders and the construction of male psychology and men's health. Some further explication of these links may be useful. I have indicated that economic change relocates men in the changing contemporary economic order and that the demands of this new order produce what might be called "new categories of men." I have also suggested that men are located in gendered, classed, and racialized hierarchies. Dominant groups of men have a continuing need to legitimate their authority in these hierarchies. As several scholars have indicated, the rhetoric of a crisis of masculinity should therefore not automatically be interpreted as a sign that men's power is abating (e.g., McMahon 1993; Brittan 1989; Hearn 1996; Robinson 2000). Instead, the crisis rhetoric is emblematic of a reconstruction and reconfirmation of men's authority in a new form.

Men are not only constituted as social categories in the economic order, but the categories also exist as representations in public discourse—as gendered discourses about men's behavior and motives. These representations form part of a moral order and lay out the moral boundaries of male identities: there exists a typification system of what constitutes a moral self (see Lamont 1992 and 2000). In some ways social science discourse could be said to have captured these representations as, for example, in the "male sex role," and health psychology constructed them as "personalities." Rather similarly, a "healthy" male identity has both in public and in scientific discourse frequently been equated with a strong male identity. Hence, a "crisis in masculinity" has been linked with a weakened and vulnerable male identity and has been seen as motivating some kind of repair. The therapeutic interventions have been headed by experts in personal "problems," and even work-related problems have in the U.S. context been interpreted as located in the individual.

In this book I have specifically looked at one type of personal problem—the coronary-prone, or Type A, personality. In the 1950s, the status strains of American men were interpreted in social science and popular discourse within the framework of sex-role theory. The foundation of this theory was the assumption that there existed a normal "healthy" sex-role identity for men. The role strains and pressures felt by Type A man became medical risk factors within the medical discourse, introduced by Friedman and Rosenman (1959), but soon psychologized into the psychological traits of Type A personality. The Type A thesis identified the coronary health problem of white middle-class men as located in their personalities.

The Type A thesis was that there existed a coronary-prone middle-class man whose behaviors and emotions signified his propensity to coronary heart problems. The medical discourse and later the scientific discourse of health psychology translated and reified these signs of men's practice into constructions called Type A, the hardy executive, and John Henryism. In my analysis I have suggested that these reifications were presented in scientific discourse as medical facts, which naturalized the social constructions of categories of men. These typifications in scientific discourse also depoliticized the underlying racial, class, and gender issues and channeled men into adopting a therapeutic approach to the perceived crisis of their authority.

I have argued that by deconstructing the typifications of personality, we can more clearly understand the underlying hierarchies of gender, race, and class inherent in the seemingly generic and unmarked personality categories. I have suggested that the typifications have served as supposedly gender-neutral tools that have both constructed men and alerted them to the status- and health-related costs of structural changes imposing new demands on and threats to dominant men in the prevailing institutional order.

I have shown that the Type A construct medicalized a certain middle-class masculinity of the 1950s—in particular, the anger, aggression, and hostility that had been the traditional display of male emotion. These emotions, the Type A thesis proposed, had health costs for these men. In contrast, the thesis of the hardy executive restored the core values of men as economic actors—men who were self-disciplined and in control. These moral qualities composed the cultural prerequisite both for the promotion of men's health and the health of the economy. The self-regulatory practices were confirmed in scientific discourse that constructed a prototype of male psychology: a man who was vulnerable to the capitalist system if he did not live up to its inner logic—the spirit of capitalism and its self-regulatory practices. The spirit of capitalism, as defined by Max Weber, demanded self-control and an internalization of an ethic that at the social level would promote the development and success of the capitalist system. Scientific discourse constructed the health costs and health-promoting traits of the American executive class as directly related to the health of the economy.

The second issue: Why did Type A achieve such a prominence in American medical and public discourse? The argument proposed in this book is that the reason for the appeal of these medical and psychological categories in public discourse is that they have reflected the values of traditional masculinity, a male role perceived as threatened. I have shown that medicine integrated the representations of certain masculinities into its language and that these representations were translated into reified categories in the scientific discourse of medicine and health psychology. In the mid-1950s, Type A became an idiom of the health costs of traditional masculinity. Type A was a culture-bound and gendered representation. It captured the strains and institutional dilemmas of American middle-class men in a certain historic and cultural setting. As a British medical anthropologist has noted, "What is most 'cultural' about this model of the origin of CHD is the content and boundaries of the model itself" (Helman 1987, 975).

The cultural image of the pioneering personality construct Type A has had a powerful appeal in American public discourse. The medical thinking on Type A resonated with a value structure that puts an emphasis on the individual. It is in this sense that the psychological interpretation of men's proneness to heart disease has been congruent with an economy in which the male executive is the major economic actor, who embodies the values of hard work, commitment to work, and the work ethic. These male-gendered work values have reflected the organizing principles of work arrangements in economies to which sociologists have given a variety of labels—for example, corporate capitalism, Fordist and post-Fordist economy, and neoliberal economy. In these kinds of market-driven economies, the moral order of work has been the moral order of the dominant groups of men. The medical thinking about Type A, the hardy executive, and John Henryism is not only about men's health, but also about the moral order and hierarchies of gender, race, and class.

The third issue: How well has psychology served to explicate men's health? Health psychology has certainly provided a way of making men aware of the health costs of a certain cultural repertoire of masculine behavior. In medical discourse Type A is a construct sanitized of any notions of men as victims of a gender order, although the concept implicitly addressed this issue. Yet, the naming of certain emotions as a health risk and an awareness of their relation to work did not perhaps so much change the men suffering from "hurry sickness" as it made them aware of preventive measures to remain healthy.

Nevertheless, the focus on certain risk factors as *men's* problem and heart disease as a killer of *men* has belittled several important aspects of this disease. The focus on men has had two consequences. First, it homogenized men and came thereby to neglect differences between men and their different rates of heart disease. The underdiagnosis and neglect of heart disease among African American men is a case in point. Second, the focus on men has made women sufferers of heart disease invisible, especially black women, who during the past fifty years have had higher death rates from heart disease than have white women, as chapter 6 shows.

The personality-focused etiological theories on CHD have promoted an individual approach to illness, and the construct of Type A personality has been part of a psychological theory of men's health. As shown in this book, Type A as a model of disease etiology is based on psychologism and methodological individualism. As defined in chapter 1, explanations taking as their departure the notion that social phenomena can be reduced to psychological phenomena adopt an approach called psychologism (Popper 1962, 88–98). This type of explanation is, furthermore, based on so-called methodological individualism, which takes its departure from the assumption that the behavior and attitudes of social groups can be reduced to the behavior and the actions of individuals (Popper 1962, 91). Collective or social phenomena are, according to this view, merely the aggregate of the actions and attitudes of single individuals, rather than the reflections of shared material conditions, experiences of the social environment, or effects of a social institution.

While representatives of public health and medical sociology have focused on different rates of heart disease in groups sharing certain demographic characteristics, health psychologists have looked at individual differences, in particular the personality predisposition related to CHD. In this enterprise, health psychologists have been very successful in influencing popular thinking about risks related to heart disease. Good examples are concepts like stress and burnout, constructed in the scientific discourse of health psychology from 1960 onwards and immediately absorbed into public discourse.

The scientific discourse of health psychology has been able to identify the cultural nerve of modern living and has provided metaphors describing and reflecting individuals' anxieties in the prevailing social and psychological space. Psychological constructs—like Type A personality—have translated the popular metaphors of the strains of modern living into scientific facts. Using the terms of C. Wright Mills (1959), it could be said that health psychology has been able to identify and name the "personal troubles" of our time and in this endeavor has aided individuals in understanding themselves as objects of self-reflection and self-diagnosis.

But the personality constructs have been presented as universal categories, unmarked by gender, class, race, and ethnicity. Still, the space described by health psychology is largely occupied by the middle class, a privileged group in the gender, racial, and economic order. This selective audience might also have been the very reason for the success of the scientific discourse of health psychology over medical sociology. Health psychology has all along addressed the plight of the middle class. The constructs of health psychology have resonated with the life situations and emotions of this health-conscious class and provided individual-level concepts and solutions. In contrast, medical and health sociologists have addressed social-level issues, generally those concerning the plight of social groups with little or no purchasing power.

Mills (1959, 8) drew a distinction between *personal troubles of milieu* and *public issues of social structure*. A division of labor in health research seems to have developed vis-à-vis these two concerns: Health psychology has constructed its scientific discourse around "personal troubles," while the scientific discourse of medical sociology has focused on "public issues." Nevertheless, medical sociologists have not been as fully successful as health psychologists in translating the respective issues into their discipline and in communicating with the public. The social and structural issues have not resonated with the values of an economic and political structure in a society that distributes resources and rewards mainly through the marketplace. Recent genetical and biosocial thinking has further confirmed this individualistic approach to health and illness.

TYPE A IN PUBLIC DISCOURSE

As chapter 4 shows, by the mid-1980s, scientific medicine had discredited the Type A hypothesis—the link between Type A behavioral pattern and CHD. But medical folklore about the Type A personality and the health hazards of this kind of personality and work behavior live on. In public discourse the tale of Type A seems still to be a medical truth, especially for a middle-aged generation.

With a stretch of imagination and of the historical allegory, it could be argued that Friedman and Rosenman in 1959 provided a health manifesto for the middle-class executive when they introduced the Type A behavioral pattern historically equivalent to the one Friedrich Engels had provided for the English working class in his exposé of the living conditions and health of that class in *The Conditions of the Working Class in England* (see Waitzkin 2000,

56–60). Both works established a new medical gaze focusing on new aspects of the etiology of deadly diseases such as CHD and tuberculosis, respectively, challenging the narrow view of medicine. Both works provided a profound analysis of the causal relationships between social structure and physical illness and the disease-producing features of the work environment. Although Friedman and Rosenman's works certainly are not the classics of social medicine and public health that Engel's work is, the central theme is the same: men's health cannot be understood without looking at men in their place of work in a market-driven economy.

It is an irony in the history of medicine that the creation of Type A in medical discourse and later in psychological discourse privatized men's health problems, while the embracing of Type A in public discourse resulted in a collective awareness of the health hazards of the work conditions of white-collar workers. Armed with a new concept, Type A, individuals could challenge the kind of work behavior and the demands set by the organization of work that both attracted and produced Type A men.

The concept Type A gave a whole generation of American middle-class men and women a language for exploring the relation between their ambitions, their competency, and the costs of achieving these goals at a time when the cultural climate described working life as full of opportunities and careers. For many, the construct of Type A was a way of making sense of the physical and emotional costs of the prevailing work ethic. Nikolas Rose has examined the rise of the modern self and characterized the impact of psychology in the following terms: "Whatever the origin of these languages of the self, they were indispensable to the ways in which we can make ourselves the objects of our reflections" (1997, 235). The construct Type A became a key language of the self for middle-class Americans. Type A provided "a grammar of the self," a psychological language and a gaze that enabled individuals to conceive of themselves both as subjects and objects in relation to their work, striving, and potential selves.

In public discourse, Type A was soon perceived as a universal trait of ambitious and career-striving individuals. In public discourse, Type A was stripped of its medical content and became a marker of a moral self. Type A has served the function of identifying what Michèle Lamont has called the moral boundary of worthy men (1992 and 2000). Type A signifies the hardworking, relentless, striving, working white-collar man who tries to prove and confirm his manliness by means of his work. Type A has become a representation of a special form of American martyrdom: it signifies a willingness to put one's body at risk in order to achieve the societally revered goals of success. The construct is composed of a set of behavioral traits associated with masculinity and is still part of the normative cultural repertoire of the United States, a culture that Kimmel calls the "manufacturing of manhood"

(1997, 157). It is ironic that as women have entered the labor force and ascended the career ladder, even they have, with some pride, described themselves as Type A people. This trend only provides further evidence of the male values embedded in the current organizational arrangement of work and management. A recent representative is Martha Stewart, who has described herself, and certainly been depicted by others, as Type A.

It was not until well into the 1990s that the American middle class took to the term *quality time* to describe their adaptation to the Type A mentality in working life, which segmented their lives between work, family, and emotions. As sociologists diagnosed it (e.g., Hochschild 1997), there was the first, second, and third shift and in between some quality time—a kind of deferred intimacy—spent with significant others.

Typification of Personalities

The alphabetical types of personalities reviewed in this book have provided a typification scheme for medicine to predict men's likelihood of getting CHD. Type A, Type C, and John Henryism have been seen as personality types related to disease-promoting traits, while Type B and hardiness have been related to a health-promoting style.

Is there a new personality type on the horizon? New alphabetical types are still emerging in public discourse. The advertising business appeals to the collective memory of Type A in American media. For example, in the spring of 2003, Bacardi took three full pages in the *New Yorker* to advertise its orange-flavored rum, the first page featuring only the question "Are you Type O?" in white lettering against a black background. In the subsequent two pages the same question is repeated in smaller print, but supported by both a longer text and a picture of what kind of man this sophisticated consumer "Type O" is. Type O man is portrayed as being in control of his life.

Currently, the idea of the hardy executive still matches the kind of man who has the cultural and moral qualities needed for surviving in the current global economy on the brink of recession. Some might be inclined to suggest that "hurry sickness" and all the behavioral signs of the Type A man of the 1950s perfectly match the behavior characteristic of a man working in the option-guided economy in the 1990s. This is a success-driven, compulsively hard-working man, who has few other interests than worldly success. As the strength of the option-guided economy is abating, this social category of men might begin to experience the same sense of loss of control and anxieties as Type A man in the 1950s.

The current rhetoric of the health crisis of men and their health disadvantage could be interpreted in the light of the current economic decline, which threatens the economic and thereby the social position of white-collar men in the current gender order. Men's health discourse can therefore be seen as a way of raising men's awareness of the future health problems of those who work in the risky zones of the current global economy.

In the 1990s, behavioral medicine launched a new personality type, Type D, in the alphabet of personalities. Type D is short for "distressed personality," a type shown to be related to cardiac disease. This personality has been characterized by negative emotions and social inhibition. Type D is emblematic of the emotional traits of a man who is not willing to disclose to himself or to others his failure as an economic actor.

It is with a sense of déjà vu that one reads Type D's Belgian promoter's early reflections on the need for more research into Type D and for personality-focused research on CHD: "It is hard to believe that personality is not related to the development and progression of disease. A major difficulty, however, concerns the definition and measurement of personality. Until these problems are resolved, inconsistent outcomes are likely in this area" (Denollet 1993, 133).

Later studies on Type D have confirmed the need "to adopt a personality approach in the early identification of those coronary patients who are at risk for emotional stress-related cardiac events" (Denollet 2000, 256). Nevertheless, the Type D personality construct has only been used by researchers in behavioral medicine and so far has not been annexed by a wider medical establishment or adopted in American public discourse.

THE PERENNIAL HEART FAILURE EPIDEMIC

In October of 2002, an editorial, "Heart Failure—An Epidemic of Uncertain Proportions," in the *New England Journal of Medicine* alerted the medical community that "we are in the midst of a proclaimed epidemic of heart failure" as measured by the mere numbers of hospitalizations, deaths, and costs of care for CHD (Redfield 2002, 1442). The editorial drew attention to an article in the same issue that presented an update from the Framingham Heart Study, showing that the incidence of heart failure has changed little among men from 1950 to the 1990s (and declined by about one-third among women) and that the rates of death after the onset of heart failure declined by about one-third in both sexes (Levy et al., 2002). The figures remind us that the cause of CHD for men is still murky, while the survival rates after the onset of heart failure have improved. The figures also confirm the epidemiological turn that took place since 1970. Around 1968, CHD mortality began to decline after decades of growth (Goldman and Cook 1984). This decline is shown in chapter 6, which documents that the death rate from heart diseases dropped by half from 1950 to 1998, although a wide health gap still exists between black and white men (table 6.1).

The editorial in the *New England Journal of Medicine* points to a paradox. Despite the falling death rates over the past forty years, there is still a heart disease epidemic lurking. Three reasons have more recently been raised. One reason is the increasing proportion of old people. Projected demographics indicate a future rise in the number of people 65 years old and older. For example, in 1960, the year following the introduction of the Type A hypothesis in medical literature, 9 percent of the American population was 65 years and over, but in 2040, 20 percent of the population will be of that age. This demographic transition will in itself produce a growing number of people with heart failure in the United States.

A second reason is the problem of obesity in American adults. In February of 2003, a special section in an issue of *Science* called this phenomenon the "obesity epidemic." This theme evokes a sense of déjà vu. Again the plight of the nation's obese is being taken to heart, as it was in the 1950s (see Berrett 1997). According to a recent National Health and Nutrition Examination Survey (NHANES), the figures for obesity in the adult population have risen to 65 percent in 1999–2000 from 56 percent a decade earlier (i.e., obesity being defined as having a body mass index greater than 25 kg/m^2) (e.g., Hill et al., 2003).

A third reason is that the issue of the onset of heart disease is still unresolved. As the editorial referred to above in the *New England Journal of Medicine* points out, there is little hope for the heart failure epidemic to end because recent data "underscore the complexity of the epidemic and our inability to understand with confidence whether—let alone why—the epidemiology of heart failure is changing" (Redfield 2002, 1444). Are there new research directions that can answer this question?

NEW RESEARCH DIRECTIONS INTO
THE PSYCHOSOCIAL DIMENSIONS OF CHD

The psychologization of Type A men set the stage for two research trends in stress research over the next thirty years. One trend was a shift in the 1980s in the focus of personality research from risk factors to health protective factors. Another trend, in the 1980s and 1990s, was a shift in the research from personal disposition to interpersonal factors and to a certain social environment as a disease-promoting factor or as a health-promoting factor. In the latter research, the concept of "psychosocial factors" has become a form of shorthand for the mediating role of emotions and the social environment and their influence on health.

In research on psychosocial factors, three different levels of concern can be identified: (1) intrapersonal factors, (2) interpersonal factors, and (3) the social environment (Weiss et al., 1990). This volume has focused on the first level—intrapersonal factors, especially personality traits as a link to CHD. Some later individual-focused research on CHD has promoted approaches that take into consideration the environment, interpreted as a form of second nature. Some of these researchers, like Stanford neurobiologist Robert Sapolsky (1994), take a critical look at modern society and its demands and examine stress-related diseases and mechanisms of coping with stress, especially the biological and psychological stress reactions that modern living produces in the body. This kind of approach harbors a notion of an archaic body that is outmoded and revolts against the "unnatural" environment of today's high technology and fast work pace (Kugelmann 1992, 34–35). Stress reveals to us the primal character of humans and the archaic body's "natural" biological reaction, also defined as the "body's own wisdom" (Freund 1982, 25). Stress reactions are therefore perceived as a "problem of corporeal hardware" (Kugelmann 1992, 42). This kind of approach has been represented by researchers whose explanatory framework is a psychophysiological reactivity model or psychoneuroimmunology (see McEwen 2000). For example, studies have looked at how the neuroendocrine system of humans affects the functioning of the immune system and, thereby, health. Research has documented the links between negative emotions and hostility—a current remnant of Type A—and hypertension (e.g., Fredrickson et al., 2000), as well as hardiness as a protective immunity shield against disease (e.g., Dolbier et al., 2001).

The second level is represented by researchers who have focused on interpersonal factors. If the former approach of the archaic body represents biological determinism, there is another that represents sociological determinism and embraces a notion of the body as in exile (Kugelmann 1992, 36–38). It is believed that modern humans have lost their traditions, common values, and a sense of meaning as the traditional tightly knit community has eroded. This explanatory framework has its theoretical roots in a Durkheimian approach that has examined how social integration and social cohesion influence mortality rates. As early as the beginning of the 1940s, Talcott Parsons reflected on how the change in the social fabric affected the health of Americans. According to him, the social isolation of the elderly from kinship, occupational, and community ties makes old age a "problem." He suggested that "through well-known psychosomatic mechanisms, the increased incidence of the disabilities of older people, such as heart disease, cancer, etc. may be at least in part attributed to this structural situation" (Parsons 1942, 616). This thesis of the link between the level of social integration or social cohesion and health has had a revival since the early 1980s. In the 1980s, concepts such as social networks and social support were seen as the kind of psychosocial buffer and health-promoting factor needed for the individual to remain healthy, even though researchers asked for clear operational definitions of these concepts in health research (e.g., Berkman 1984; Berkman et al., 2000).

The concepts of social networks and social support have focused on the relationship between the individual and the primary group, measured by a person's social networks. In the 1990s, the same theme continued, but now with a focus on the community, especially the sense of community, trust, and social cohesion that were assumed to explain social differences in health. This community-level analysis has developed into the so-called social-capital theory.

Since the mid-1990s, Robert Putnam's essay and later book *Bowling Alone* (1995 and 2000) have been frequently cited references for the origin of this theory. Putnam's allegory of the atomized individual who is bowling alone captures the old theme of a longing for a tight community and a sense of belonging. Putnam argues that the American social fabric is fragmented because of a whole set of demographic, social, and technological changes and a decline of civic organizations in the United States. The consequence is a "growing social-capital deficit," which, he suggests, "threatens educational performance, safe neighborhoods, equitable tax collection, democratic responsiveness, everyday honesty, and even our health and happiness" (Putnam 2000, 367).

This theme of the lost small-town community is a perpetual concern on the mental map of Americans. The loss of the golden age of American small-town life has been expressed in past populist movements (Hofstadter 1955) and in American popular science—for example, in David Riesman's *The Lonely Crowd* (1950), although the tight grip of this small-town life on its men has also been the target of satire in American literature, as exemplified in Sinclair Lewis's classic *Babbitt* (1950).

The thesis about the link between social capital and health has been put to the test in a number of different kinds of studies. The debate has centered around the effect of a decline in social cohesion on health, a theme reintroduced by the British researcher Richard Wilkinson (1996), who suggested that social inequality influences social relationships and ultimately health and that the link to health is psychosocial. It is assumed that social inequality influences health through an individual's perception of his or her location in the social hierarchy. This theme has been further developed by, for example, Harvard School of Public Health–based Ichiro Kawachi and Bruce P. Kennedy, who declared: "A large gap between rich people and poor people leads to higher mortality through the breakdown of social cohesion" (1997, 1037).

More lately the concept of social capital has captured a wide variety of ideological concerns about the relationship between social integration or social cohesion and health. Researchers of a communitarian stripe see a restoration of a sense of community and voluntary organizations as the social capital that will improve both individual and social health. Others who profess libertarian views give social capital a more market-oriented meaning. They perceive the restoration of trust as the necessary normative and social infrastructure for both the workings of the society and the market. A society based on trust has the kind of social capital for not only the workings of the society, but of capitalism as well (e.g., Fukuyama 1995, 27). In the twenty-first century the latter views have been associated with a neoliberal doctrine of how society should be organized. The economic actor has become the prime social actor, who through the market is assumed to gain full agency (Lemke 2001).

Here the social thinking in the 1970s seems to be recycled: at that time the introduction of the consumer in political life was seen as an appropriate corrective measure for any imbalance of power. The economic allegory was even then misplaced, because the term *consumer* privileged the middle class with its purchasing power. The term *consumer*—like the current term *social capital*—may tend to render the poor and the imbalances in power invisible. In both cases the use of economic terminology to explain social phenomena obfuscates the structural and political aspects of the phenomena.

In contrast to the foregoing cultural interpretation of social disorganization, there is a material one, too. This explanation suggests that structural and material causes of inequalities, rather than merely perceptions of inequality, affect health (e.g., Pearce and Smith 2003, 126). Such a critical examination of the effects of social disorganization is exemplified in the research looking at inner cities and the high prevalence of cardiovascular disease factors among their poor, predominantly black residents (e.g., Diez-Roux et al., 1999). It has been argued that people living in disadvantaged neighborhoods are faced with the stresses brought by crime, fear, and a noxious environment that impairs their health (Ross and Mirowsky 2001; Cohen et al., 2003). This kind of research suggests that socioeconomic conditions are the primary origins of the racial stratification of health (e.g., the racial differences in the prevalence of hypertension, heart disease, and stroke) (Hayward et al., 2000, 921).

In a more conservative political climate today, terms like *trust* and *social capital* have become a way of analyzing the "health" of society. The term *social capital* transforms capital into an asset in social life: Individuals should be rich in social capital that guarantees that they get ahead in a competitive society and economy. At the community level, social capital is seen as a precondition for economic capital and for economic growth. In his critique of the term *social capital*, Vicente Navarro laments such a view of society because "the purpose of all social action is reduced to accumulating more capital so that the individual can compete better" (2002, 427).

As representatives of the materialist critique of the social-capital thesis on health suggest, a lack of social cohesion can be a product of the social inequality and social fragmentation of society caused by the competitiveness of laissez-faire capitalism and an undermining of the welfare state. As Coburn suggests, "There does seem a contradiction between an increasing emphasis on social capital and social cohesion under regimes which are actually undermining these processes" (2000, 143). This neo-Marxist perspective has been put to the test in a study by Charles Muntaner et al. on the link between health variables and income inequality (2002). The research group concludes that the incorporation of class, race, and gender economics and politics is needed in order to show the limitations of social capital and similar psychosocial models (Muntaner et al., 2002, 655). Similar voices are heard from British researchers who deplore the romanticized picture of the traditional community in the social-capital theory. Furthermore, the theory offers little in the way of effective intervention. As Pearce and Smith suggest, it sets unrealistic expectations of community involvement and resources and diverts attention from the health effects of macrolevel social and economic policies (2003, 128).

The third level of research on psychosocial factors and health involves the social environment and has its followers in the area of working-life research and occupational health (e.g., Karasek and Theorell 1990). In this research, the extent of control over work has served as an important factor for interpreting workers' stress-related behavior and health. This research has used a psychological framework and become a genre called job stress research. A couple of models have influenced the research, of which the person-environment-fit model and the demand-control model today constitute the classics. The person-environment-fit model was introduced and tested by a research group at the University of Michigan, Ann Arbor (Harrison 1978; French et al., 1982). This model postulates that an imbalance between a person's abilities and the demands of the job will result in stress. Another model is the demand-control model, which suggests that jobs characterized by high demands and low job control will be stressful (Karasek 1979).

Both models were originally tested on a sample of only male workers. Karasek argued that the inclusion of women in studies of job stress would complicate the research design, because, as he stated, "the relationship between work and mental health status for women is often complicated by the additional demand of housework" (1979, 289). The assumption was that a study of males only guaranteed the validity of the measures because an examination of men at work would measure only their thoughts and behavior at work. Still, the implications of the findings of the job-demand model, and person-environment-fit model as well, were for a long time applied to all workers. Subsequent research has introduced women and a variety of health problems into the testing of the models (e.g., Karasek and Theorell 1990; Kasl 1996; Peter and Siegrist 1997; Bosma et al., 1998).

Why Is Gender Invisible in These New Research Directions?

The three new research directions on psychosocial factors and illness reviewed above can be rephrased as portraying the archaic body, the body in exile, and the body at work. Each of the three portrayals captures a specific causal framework.

First, the notion of the archaic body rests on thinking represented by biological reductionism. This perspective attributes prime explanatory power to biological factors. This thinking has had a revival in recent genetic explanations: We are the outcomes of our genes (Rothman 1998; Conrad 2000). In these explanations, the archaic body looks surprisingly familiar: it is the male body, even though the transhistorical and culturally universal and unmarked generic body is presented as *the* biological reality—as nature. As chapter 2 shows, in men's health discourses we find that the rightist streams of thinking on men's health and the health costs of a tarnished masculinity are based on this explanatory framework. This notion of stress and health renders cultural and social practices invisible, while it constructs and confirms a homogenized and essentialist notion of the male body and men's health.

Second, the notion of the body as in exile adopts a view that reflects sociological reductionism. According to this view, individuals are blank slates who are programmed by culture and social norms. The attitudes and behaviors of individuals are explained by social factors alone. If the social programming abates, as measured by a weakening social consensus and trust and social integration, it is assumed that not only social, but individual, health deteriorates. This view provides a romanticized picture of a Gemeinschaft-like, preindustrial type of society, where social distances were assumed to be minor and common rituals and traditions confirmed people's place in the traditional order. Again this social order also seems very familiar from a gender perspective: it is a traditional patriarchal society that provides little cultural and social space for different types of masculinities.

Third, a focus on the body at work is represented by workplace studies that suggest that working-life research captures an almost naturalistic context for a study of men in action. There is an underlying notion of the working man as hero in these studies. Either he is a blue-collar hero fighting against unnatural working conditions, or he is the manager hero striving by his rational actions to strengthen the sound structure of not only the workplace, but also of the economic order. In short, the naturalistic context of work provides a laboratory-like setting for the study of man as a cultural and social being willing to put his body at risk to prove his healthy status as a man. This thinking is characterized by a psychological reductionism: models of social behavior are developed from psychological factors (e.g., it is assumed that motives are based on essential needs and psychological reactions to such needs). The naturalistic context of work provides, therefore, an opportunity to unravel man's essential nature and his natural reactions to blocked agency and full agency. In the language used in this book, the assumption underlying workplace studies is that they offer an opportunity to study wounded and healthy masculinities.

The research referred to above has for most part not looked at the role of gender as the social context of how the individual lives and experiences his or her life situation and what the social consequences of gender are for each gender. The social epidemiology research tradition has looked at sex differences, but it has generally taken a variable approach and operationalized gender as a dichotomous variable. This focus on sex differences in health outcomes does not problematize the differences in health as part of the social conditions of a gender order. The sex-difference research on health is often based on sex-role theory, which frames how the health differences are understood and explained (Annandale and Hunt 2000). The need to understand the gendered context of health outcomes has been privileged by scholars who have called for a gender-informed and gender-relations approach (Schofield et al., 2000; Sabo 2000), as well as a gender-comparative approach to health (Annandale and Hunt 2000). Both emphasize the need to examine the gender order and relations between genders in research on men's and women's health and the need to address the diversities of masculinity and femininity in the current economic and social order.

Health is not randomly distributed in society, but socially structured, and a preventive approach should consider how health is socially structured. Research on men's health from a gender-sensitive perspective is a research direction that is a challenge to promote. Efforts to unveil the gendered, classed, and racialized character of men's health would make transparent the seemingly unmarked character of the dominant groups of men. Using such a framework would provide new insights into the health patterns of different groups of men and women.

Bibliography

Abbott, Andrew. 1988. *The systems of professions*. Chicago: Univ. of Chicago Press.

American Heart Association. 2003. *Cardiovascular disease statistics*, www .americanheart.org (accessed February 13, 2003).

American Sociological Association. 2003. *The importance of collecting data and doing social scientific research on race*. Washington, DC: American Sociological Association.

Angell, Marcia. 1985. Disease as a reflection of the psyche. *New England Journal of Medicine* 312:1570–1572.

Annandale, Ellen, and Kate Hunt. 2000. Gender inequalities in health: Research at the crossroads. In *Gender inequalities in health*, edited by Ellen Annandale and Kate Hunt, 1–35. Buckingham, U.K.: Open Univ. Press.

Armstrong, David. 1990. Use of the genealogical method in the exploration of chronic illness: A research note. *Social Science and Medicine* 30:1225–1227.

———. 1995. The rise of surveillance medicine. *Sociology of Health and Illness* 17:393–404.

Aronowitz, Robert A. 1998. *Making sense of illness: Science, society and disease*. Cambridge: Cambridge Univ. Press.

Barnett, Elisabeth, Donna L. Armstrong, and Michele L. Casper. 1999. Evidence of increasing coronary heart disease mortality among black men of lower class. *Annals of Epidemiology* 9:464–471.

Bartley, Mel. 1985. Coronary heart disease and the public health, 1850–1983. *Sociology of Health and Illness* 7:289–313.

Berger, Peter L., and Thomas Luckman. 1967. *The social construction of reality: A treatise in the sociology of knowledge*. Garden City, NY: Doubleday.

Berkman, Lisa F. 1984. Assessing the physical health effects of social networks and social support. *Annual Review of Public Health* 5:413–432.

Berkman, Lisa F., Thomas Glass, Ian Brisette, and Teresa E. Seeman. 2000. From social integration to health: Durkheim in the new millennium. *Social Science and Medicine* 51:843–857.

Berrett, Jesse. 1997. Feeding the organization man: Diet and masculinity in postwar America. *Journal of Social History* 30:805–825.

Billman, Carol. 1986. *The secret of the Stratemeyer Syndicate: Nancy Drew, the Hardy Boys, and the million dollar fiction factory.* New York: The Ungar Publishing Company.

Bordo, Susan. 2000. *The male body: A new look at men in public and private.* New York: Farrar, Straus and Giroux.

Bortner, Rayman W. 1969. A short rating scale as a potential measure of pattern A behavior. *Journal of Chronic Disease* 22:87–91.

Bosma, Hans, Richard Peter, and Johannes Siegrist. 1998. Two alternative job stress models and the risk of coronary heart disease. *American Journal of Public Health* 88:68–74.

Boston Women's Health Collective. 1973. *Our bodies, ourselves: A book by and for women.* New York: Simon & Schuster.

Brandt, Allan M. 2000. Racism and research: The case of the Tuskegee Syphilis experiment. In *Tuskegee's truth: Rethinking the Tuskegee Syphilis Study*, edited by Susan M. Reverby, 15–33. Chapel Hill: Univ. of North Carolina Press.

Brittan, Arthur. 1989. *Masculinity and power.* Oxford: Blackwell.

Brooks, Gary R. 2001. Masculinity and men's mental health. *Journal of American College Health* 49:285–297.

Broverman, Inge K., Donald M. Broverman, Frank E. Clarkson, Paul S. Rosenkrantz, and Susan R. Vogel. 1970. Sex-role stereotypes and clinical judgements of mental health. *Journal of Consulting and Clinical Psychology* 34:1–7.

Buck, Rodger L. 1961. Behavioral scientists in schools of medicine. *Journal of Health and Human Behavior* 2:59–64.

Bush, George W. 2002. Transcript of president's address calling for new era of corporate integrity. *New York Times*, 10 July 2002, C4.

Butler, Judith. 1993. *Bodies that matter: On the discursive limits of "sex."* London: Routledge.

Byrd, W. Michael, and Linda A. Clayton. 2002. *An American health dilemma.* Vol. 2. of *Race, medicine, and health care in the United States, 1900–2000.* New York: Routledge.

Carby, Hazel V. 1998. *Race men.* Cambridge, MA: Harvard Univ. Press.

Case Robert B., Stanley S. Heller, Nan B. Case, Arthur J. Moss, and the Multicenter Post-Infarction Research Group. 1985. Type A behavior and survival after myocardial infarction. *New England Journal of Medicine* 312:737–741.

Cassell, Eric J. 1986. Ideas in conflict: The rise and fall (and rise and fall) of new views of disease. *Daedalus* 115(2): 19–41.

Chesler, Phyllis. 1989. *Women and madness.* New York: Harcourt Brace Jovanovich. (Orig. pub. 1972.)

Coburn, David. 2000. Income inequality, social cohesion and the health status of populations: The role of neo-liberalism. *Social Science and Medicine* 51:135–146.

Cohen, Deborah A., Karen Mason, Ariane Bedimo, Richard Scribner, Victoria Basolo, and Thomas Farley. 2003. Neighborhood physical conditions and health. *American Journal of Public Health* 93:467–471.

Connell, R. W. 1987. *Gender and power: Society, the person and sexual politics*. Palo Alto, CA: Stanford Univ. Press.

———. 1995. *Masculinities*. Berkeley: Univ. of California Press.

———. 2000. *The Men and the boys*. Berkeley: Univ. of California Press.

Conrad, Peter. 1992. Medicalization and social control. *Annual Review of Sociology* 18:209–232.

———. 2000. Medicalization, genetics, and human problems. In *Handbook of medical sociology*, edited by Cloe E. Bird, Peter Conrad, and Allen M. Fremont, 5th ed., 322–333. Upper Saddle River, NJ: Prentice Hall.

Contrada, J. Richard, Howard Leventhal, and Ann O'Leary. 1990. Personality and health. In *Handbook of personality: Theory and research*, edited by Lawrence A. Pervin, 638–669. New York: Guildford Press.

Cooley, Charles Horton. 1902. *The two major works of Charles H. Cooley: Social organization, human nature and the social order.* Repr., Glencoe, IL: Free Press, 1956.

Corti, Maria-Chiara, Jack M. Guralnik, Luigi, Ferrucci et al. 1999. Evidence for a black-white crossover in all-cause and coronary heart disease mortality in an older population: The North Carolina EPESE. *American Journal of Public Health* 89:308–314.

Courtenay, Will H. 2000. Constructions of masculinity and their influence on men's well-being: A theory of gender and health. *Social Science and Medicine* 50:1385–1401.

Courtenay, Will H., and Richard P. Keeling. 2000. Men, gender and health: Toward an interdisciplinary approach. *Journal of American College Health* 48:243–246.

Crawford, Robert. 1980. Healthism and the medicalization of everyday life. *International Journal of Health Services* 10:365–388.

Danziger, Kurt. 1990. *Constructing the subject: Historical origins of psychological research.* Cambridge: Cambridge Univ. Press.

———. 1997. *Naming the mind: How psychology found its language.* London: Sage.

Davis, Kathy. 2002. "A dubious equality": Men, women and cosmetic surgery. *Body and Society* 8:49–65.

Denollet, Johan. 1993. Biobehavioral research on coronary heart disease: Where is the person? *Journal of Behavioral Medicine* 16:115–141.

———. 1998. Personality and coronary heart disease: The Type-D scale-16 (DS16). *Annals of Behavioral Medicine* 20:209–215.

———. 2000. Type D Personality: A Potential Risk Factor Refined. *Journal of Psychosomatic Research* 49:255–266.

Denollet, Johan, and Guus Van Heck. 2001. Psychological risk factors in heart disease: What Type D personality is (not) about. *Journal of Psychosomatic Research* 51:465–468.

Denollet, Johan, Stanislaus U. Sys, and Dirk L. Brutsaert. 1995. Personality and mortality after myocardial infarction. *Psychosomatic Medicine* 57:582–591.

Denollet, Johan, Stanislaus U. Sys, Natalie Stroobant, Hans Rombouts, Thierry C. Gillebert, and Dirk L. Brutsaert. 1996. Personality as Independent predictor of long-term mortality in patients with coronary heart disease. *Lancet* 347:417–421.

Devereux, George. 1964. Two types of modal personality models. In *Personality and social systems*, edited by Neil J. Smelser and William T. Smelser, 22–32. New York: John Wiley & Sons.

Diez-Roux, Ana, Mary E. Northridge, Alfredo Morabia, Mary T. Bassett, and Steven Shea. 1999. Prevalence and social correlates of cardiovascular disease risk factors in Harlem. *American Journal of Public Health* 89:302–307.

Dimsdale, Joel E. 1988. A perspective on Type A behavior and coronary disease. *New England Journal of Medicine* 318:110–112.

Dixon, Franklin W. 1927. *The tower treasure*. New York: Grosset & Dunlap, Inc.

——. 1928. *The missing chums*. New York: Grosset & Dunlap, Inc.

——. 1947. *The phantom freighter*. New York: Grosset & Dunlap Publishers.

——. 2002. *The Hardy boys' guide to life*. New York: Simon & Schuster.

Dolbier, Christyn L., Robert R. Cocke, Jenn A. Leiferman, Mary A. Steinhardt, Steven J. Schapiro, Pramod N. Nehete, Jaine E. Perlman, and Jagannadha Sastry. 2001. Differences in functional immune responses of high vs. low hardy healthy individuals. *Journal of Behavioral Medicine* 24:219–229.

Doyal, Leslie. 2001. Sex, gender and health: The need for a new approach. *British Medical Journal* 323:1061–1063.

Drake, St. Clair, and Horace R. Cayton. 1945. *Black metropolis: A study of Negro life in a northern city*. New York: Harcourt Brace & Company.

Dyson, Michael Erik. 1996. *Between God and gangsta rap: Bearing witness to black culture*. New York: Oxford Univ. Press.

Eaker, Elaine D., Suzanne G. Haynes, and Manning Feinleib. 1983. Spouse behavior and coronary heart disease in men: Prospective results from the Framingham Heart Study. II: Modification of risk in Type A husbands according to the social and psychological status of their wives. *American Journal of Epidemiology* 118:23–41.

Edwards, Jeffrey R. 1991. The measurement of Type A behavior pattern: An assessment of criterion-oriented validity, content validity, and construct validity. In *Personality and stress: Individual differences in the stress process*, edited by Cary L. Cooper and Roy Payne, 151–180. New York: John Wiley & Sons.

Ehrenreich, Barbara. 1983. *The hearts of men: American dreams and the flight from commitment*. Garden City, NY: Anchor Press/Doubleday.

Eichler, Margrit. 1980. *The double standard: A feminist critique of feminist social science*. London: Croom Helm.

Erikson, Kai T. 1966. *The wayward Puritans: A study in the sociology of deviance*. New York: John Wiley & Sons.

Foucault, Michel. 1975. *The birth of the clinic: An archaelogy of medical perception*. New York: Vintage Books.

——. 1988. Technologies of the self. In *Technologies of the self*, edited by Luther M. H. Martin, Huck Gutman, and Patrick H. Hutton, 16–49. Amherst: Univ. of Massachusetts Press.

Fred, Herbert L., and Ramesh Hariharan. 2002. To be B or not to be B—Is that the question? *Texas Heart Institute* 29:1–2.

Fredrickson, Barbara L., Kimberly E. Maynard, Michael J. Helms, Thomas L. Haney, Ilene C. Siegler, and John C. Barefoot. 2000. Hostility predicts magnitude and duration of blood pressure response to anger. *Journal of Behavioral Medicine* 23:229–243.

French, John R. P., Jr., Robert D. Caplan, and R. van Harrison. 1982. *The mechanism of job stress and strain.* New York: John Wiley & Sons.

Freund, Peter E. S. 1982. *The civilized body: Social domination, control, and health.* Philadelphia: Temple University Press.

Friedman, Howard S. 1990. Where is the disease-prone personality? Conclusion and future direction. In *Personality and disease*, edited by Howard S. Friedman, 283–292. New York: John Wiley.

Friedman, Howard S., and Stephanie Booth-Kewley. 1987. The "disease-prone personality": A meta-analytic view of the construct. *American Psychologist* 42:539–555.

Friedman, Meyer. 1977. Type A behavior pattern: Some of its pathophysiological components. *Bulletin of the New York Academy of Medicine* 53:593–604.

Friedman, Meyer, and Ray H. Rosenman. 1959. Association of specific overt behavior pattern with blood and cardiovascular findings. *Journal of the American Medical Association* 169:1286–1296.

———. 1960. Overt behavior pattern in coronary disease. *Journal of the American Medical Association* 173:1320–1326.

———. 1974. *Type A behavior and your heart.* New York: Alfred A. Knopf.

Friedman, Meyer, Ray H. Rosenman, and Vernice Carroll. 1958. Changes in the serum cholesterol and blood clotting time in men subjected to cyclic variation of occupational stress. *Circulation* 17:852–861.

Friedman, Meyer, and Diane Ulmer. 1984. *Treating Type A behavior and your heart.* New York: Alfred A. Knopf.

Fukuyama, Francis. 1995. *Trust: The social virtues and the creation of prosperity.* New York: Free Press.

Fullilove, Mindy Tompson. 1998. Comment: Abandoning "race" as a variable in public health research: An idea whose time has come. *American Journal of Public Health* 88:1297–1298.

Funk, Steven C. 1992. Hardiness: A review of theory and research. *Health Psychology* 11:335–345.

Funk, Steven C., and Kent B. Houston. 1987. A critical analysis of the hardiness scale's validity and utility. *Journal of Personality and Social Psychology* 53:572–578.

Gerth, Hans, and C. Wright Mills. 1954. *Character and social structure: The psychology of social institutions.* London: Routledge & Kegan Paul.

Giddens, Anthony. 1986. *The constitution of society: Outline of the theory of structuration.* Berkeley: Univ. of California Press.

———. 1991. *Modernity and self-identity: Self and society in the late modern age.* Cambridge, U.K.: Polity Press.

Gillum, Richard F. 1996. The epidemiology of cardiovascular disease in black americans. *New England Journal of Medicine* 335(21): 1597–1598.

Gillum, Richard F., and Kuo Chang Liu. 1984. Coronary heart disease mortality in united states blacks, 1940–1978: Trends and unanswered questions. *American Heart Journal* 108:728–732.

Glass, David C. 1977. *Behavior patterns, stress, and coronary disease*. Hillsdale, NJ: Lawrence Erlbaum Associates Publishers.

Goldman, Lee, and E. Francis Cook. 1984. The decline in ischemic heart disease mortality rates: An analysis of the comparative effects of medical interventions and changes in lifestyle. *Annals of Internal Medicine* 101:825–836.

Harrell, Jules P., Sadiki Hall, and James Taliaferro. 2003. Physiological responses to racism and discrimination: An assessment of the evidence. *American Journal of Public Health* 93:243–248.

Harris, Richard. 1969. *The sacred trust*. Baltimore: Penguin Books.

Harrison, James, James Chin, and Thomas Ficarrotto. 1989. Warning: Masculinity may be dangerous to your health. In *Men's Lives*, edited by Michael S. Kimmel and Michael A. Messner, 246–309. New York: Macmillan Publishing Company.

Harrison, R. van. 1978. Person-environment fit and job stress. In *Stress at work*, edited by Cary L. Cooper and Roy Payne, 175–209. New York: Wiley.

Harvey, David. 1989. The condition of postmodernity: An enquiry into the origins of cultural change. Cambridge, MA: Blackwell.

Haynes, Suzanne G., Sol Levine, Norman Scotch, Manning Feinleib, and William B. Kannel. 1978a. The relationship of psychosocial factors to coronary heart disease in the Framingham Study: I. Methods and risk factors. *American Journal of Epidemiology* 107:362–383.

Haynes, Suzanne G., Manning Feinleib, Sol Levine, Norman Scotch, and William B. Kannel. 1978b. The relationship of psychosocial factors to coronary heart disease in the Framingham Study: II. Prevalence of coronary heart disease. *American Journal of Epidemiology* 107:384–402.

Haynes, Suzanne G., Manning Feinleib, and William B. Kannel. 1980. The relationship of psychosocial factors to coronary heart disease in the Framingham Study: III. Eight-year incidence of coronary heart disease. *American Journal of Epidemiology* 111:37–58.

Haynes, Suzanne G., Elaine D. Eaker, and Manning Feinleib. 1983. Spouse behavior and coronary heart disease in men: Prospective results from the Framingham Heart Study. I: Concordance of risk factors and the relationship of psychosocial status to coronary incidence. *American Journal of Epidemiology* 118:1–22.

Hayward, Mark D., Eileen M. Crimmins, Toni P. Miles, and Yu Yang. 2000. The significance of socioeconomic status in explaining the racial gap in chronic health conditions. *American Sociological Review* 65:910–930.

Hearn, Jeff. 1996. Deconstructing the dominant: Making the one(s) the other(s). *Organization* 3:611–626.

———. 1998. Theorizing men and men's theorizing: Varieties of discursive practices in men's theorizing of men. *Theory and Society* 27:781–816.

Helgeson, Vicki S. 1995. Masculinity, men's roles, and coronary heart disease. In *Men's health and illness: Gender, power, and the body*, edited by Donald Sabo and David Frederick Gordon, 68–104. Thousand Oaks, CA: Sage.

Helman, Cecil G. 1987. Heart disease and the cultural construction of time: The Type A behaviour pattern as a Western culture-bound syndrome. *Social Science and Medicine* 25:969–979.

Hemingway, Harry, and Michael Marmot. 1999. Psychosocial factors in the aetiology and prognosis of coronary heart disease: Systematic review of prospective cohort studies. *BMJ* 318:1460–1467.

Hill, James O., Holly R. Wyatt, George W. Reed, and John C. Peters. 2003. Obesity and the environment: Where do we go from here? *Science* 299:853–855.

Hochschild, Arlie Russel. 1997. *The time bind: When work becomes home and home becomes work*. New York: Metropolitan Books.

Hofstadter, Richard. 1955. *The age of reform*. New York: Vintage.

Hughes, Everett C. 1945. Dilemmas and contradictions of status. *American Journal of Sociology* 50:353–359.

Hull, Jay G., Ronald R. Van Treuren, and Suzanne Virnelli. 1987. Hardiness and health: A critique and alternative approach. *Journal of Personality and Social Psychology* 53:518–530.

James, Sherman A. 1984a. Socioeconomic influences on coronary heart disease in black populations. *American Heart Journal* 108(3):669–672.

———. 1984b. Coronary heart disease in black Americans: Suggestions for research on psychosocial factors. *American Heart Journal* 108(3):833–838.

———. 1994. John Henryism and the health of African-Americans. *Culture, Medicine and Psychiatry* 18:163–182.

James, Sherman A., Sue A. Harnett, and William D. Kalsbeek. 1983. John Henryism and blood pressure: Differences among black men. *Journal of Behavioral Medicine* 6:259–278.

James, Sherman A., Andrea Z. LaCroix, David G. Kleinbaum, and David S. Strogatz. 1984. John Henryism and blood pressure differences among black men. II. The role of occupational stressors. *Journal of Behavioral Medicine* 7:259–275.

James, Sherman A., David S. Strogatz, Steven B. Wing, and Diane L. Lamsey. 1987. Socioeconomic status, John Henryism, and hypertension in blacks and whites. *American Journal of Epidemiology* 126:664–673.

James, Sherman A., Nora L. Keenan, David S. Strogatz, Steven R. Browning, and Joanne M. Garrett. 1992. Socioeconomic status, John Henryism, and blood pressure in black adults. *American Journal of Epidemiology* 135:59–67.

Jefferson, Tony. 1998. Muscle, "hard men" and "Iron" Mike Tyson: Reflections on desire, anxiety and the embodiment of masculinity. *Body and Society* 4:77–98.

Jenkins, C. David. 1966. Components of the coronary-prone behavior pattern: Their relation to silent myocardial infarction and blood lipids. *Journal of Chronic Disease* 19:599–609.

Jenkins, C. David, S. J. Zyzanski, and Ray H. Rosenman. 1979. *Manual for the Jenkins Activity Survey*. New York: Psychological Corporation.

Johnson, Deidre. 1993. *Edward Stratemeyer and the Stratemeyer Syndicate*. New York: Twayne Publishers.

Johnson, Ernest H., and Charles D. Spielberger. 1992. Assessment of the experience, expression, and control of anger in hypertension research. In *Personality, elevated blood pressure, and essential hypertension*, edited by Ernest H. Johnson, W. Doyle Gentry, and Steve Julius, 3–24. Washington, DC: Hemisphere Publishing Corporation.

Johnson, Katarina W., Gerlad H. Payne, and Richard F. Gillum, eds. 1984. Special issue on coronary heart disease in black populations. *American Heart Journal* 108(3), Part 2.

Jones, Paul A. (with Angela Mitchell). 1993. *The black health library guide to heart disease and hypertension.* New York: Henry Holt and Company.

Kaplan, Berton H. 1992. Social health and the forgiving heart: The Type B story. *Journal of Behavioral Medicine* 15:3–14.

Karasek, Robert A. 1979. Job Demands, job decision latitude, and mental strain: Implications for job redesign. *Administrative Science Quarterly* 24:285–308.

Karasek, Robert, and Töres Theorell. 1990. *Healthy work: Stress, productivity and the reconstruction of working life.* New York: Basic Books.

Kasl, Stanislav V. 1984. Social and psychological factors in the etiology of coronary heart disease in black populations: An exploration of research needs. *American Heart Journal* 108:660–669.

———. 1996. Influence of the work environment on cardiovascular health: A historical, conceptual, and methodological perspective. *Journal of Occupational Health Psychology* 1:42–56.

Kawachi, Ichiro, and Bruce P. Kennedy. 1997. Health and social cohesion: Why care about income inequality? *BMJ* 314:1037–1040.

Keil, Julian E., and Donald E. Saunders. 1991. Urban and rural differences in cardiovascular disease in blacks. In *Cardiovascular diseases in blacks*, edited by Elijah Saunders, 17–28. Philadelphia: F. A. Davis Company.

Keil, Julian E., C. Boyd Loadholt, Martin C. Weinrich, S. Hope Sandifer, and Edwin Boyle. 1984. Incidence of coronary heart disease in blacks in Charleston, South Carolina. *American Heart Journal* 108:779–786.

Keil, Julian E., H. A. Tyroler, and Peter C. Gazes. 1991. Predictors of coronary heart disease in blacks. In *Cardiovascular Diseases in Blacks*, edited by Elijah Saunders, 227–239. Philadelphia: F. A. Davis Company.

Keil, Julian E., Susan E. Sutherland, Rebecca G. Knapp et al. 1993. Mortality rates and risk factors for coronary heart disease in black compared with white men and women. *New England Journal of Medicine* 329:73–78.

Keil, Julian E., Susan E. Sutherland, and Curtis G. Hames et al. 1995. Coronary disease mortality and risk factors in black and white men: Results from the combined Charleston, SC, and Evans County, Georgia, heart studies. *Archives of Internal Medicine* 155:1521–1527.

Keith, Robert Allen. 1966. Personality and coronary heart disease: A review. *Journal of Chronic Disease* 19:1231–1243.

Kimmel, Michael S. 1997. *Manhood in America: A cultural history.* New York: Free Press.

———. 2000. *The gendered society.* New York: Oxford Univ. Press.

Kimmel, Michael S., and Michael Kaufman. 1995. Weekend warriors: The new men's movement. In *The politics of manhood*, edited by Michael S. Kimmel, 15–43. Philadelphia: Temple Univ. Press.

Kismaric, Carole, and Marvin Heiferman. 1998. *The mysterious case of Nancy Drew and the Hardy boys.* New York: Simon & Schuster.

Klinger, Diane, Robbya Green-Weir, David Nerenz, Suzanne Havstad, Howard S. Rosman, Leonard Cetner, Samir Shah, Frances Wimbush, and Steven Borzak. 2002. Perceptions of chest pain by race. *American Heart Journal* 144:58–59.

Kluckhohn, Clyde. 1949. *Mirror for man.* Greenwich, CT: A Fawcett Premier Book.

Kobasa, Suzanne. 1979. Stressful life events, personality, and health: An inquiry into hardiness. *Journal of Personality and Social Psychology* 37:1–11.

Kobasa, Suzanne C., Salvatore R. Maddi, and Sheila Courington. 1981. Personality and constitution as mediators in the stress-illness relationship. *Journal of Health and Social Behavior* 22:368–378.

Kobasa, Suzanne C., Salvatore R. Maddi, and Stephen Kahn, S. 1982. Hardiness and health: A prospective study. *Journal of Personality and Social Psychology* 42:168–177.

Kobasa, Suzanne C., Salvatore R. Maddi, and Marc A. Zola. 1983. Type A and hardiness. *Journal of Behavioral Medicine* 6:41–51.

Koos, Earl Lomon. 1954. *The health in Regionville.* New York: Columbia Univ. Press.

Krause, Eliott A. 1973. Health planning as a managerial ideology. *International Journal of Health Services* 3:445–463.

Krieger, Nancy. 2000. Refiguring 'race': Epidemiology, racialized biology, and biological expressions of race relations. *International Journal of Health Services* 30:211–216.

Kugelmann, Robert. 1992. *Stress: The nature and history of engineered grief.* Westport, CT: Praeger.

Kumanyika, Shiriki, and Lucile L. Adams-Campbell. 1991. Obesity, diet, and psychosocial factors contributing to cardiovascular disease in blacks. In *Cardiovascular diseases in blacks*, edited by Elijah Saunders, 47–73. Philadelphia: F. A. Davis Company.

Lamont, Michèle. 1992. *Money, morals, and manners: The culture of the French and American upper-middle class.* Chicago: Univ. of Chicago Press.

———. 2000. *The dignity of working men: Morality and boundaries of race, class, and immigration.* Cambridge, MA: Harvard Univ. Press.

Lancet. 2001. Time for creative thinking about men's health. *Lancet* 357(9271):1813.

Latour, Bruno. 1999. *Pandora's hope: Essays on the reality of science studies.* Cambridge, MA: Harvard Univ. Press.

Lemke, Thomas. 2001. "The birth of bio-politics": Michel Foucault's lecture at the Collège de France on neo-liberal governmentality. *Economy and Society* 30:109–207.

Levine, Lawrence W. 1977. *Black culture and black consciousness: Afro-American folk thought from slavery to freedom.* New York: Oxford Univ. Press.

Levy, Daniel, Satish Kenchaiah, Martin G. Larson et al. 2002. Long-term trends in the incidence of and survival with heart failure. *New England Journal of Medicine* 347:1397–1402.

Lewis, Sinclair. 1950. *Babbitt.* New York: Harcourt, Brace & World.

Lorber, Judith. 1993. Believing is seeing: Biology as ideology. *Gender and Society* 7:568–581.

———. 1994. *Paradoxes of gender.* New Haven, CT: Yale Univ. Press.

———. 2000. Using gender to undo gender: A feminist degendering movement. *Feminist Theory* 1:79–95.

Lorber, Judith, and Lisa Jean Moore. 2002. *Gender and the social construction of illness.* 2nd ed. Walnut Creek, CA: AltaMira Press.

Lunbeck, Elizabeth. 1998. American psychiatrists and the modern man, 1900 to 1920. *Men and Masculinities* 1:58–86.

Lupton, Deborah. 1997. Foucault and the medicalization critique. In *Foucault: Health and medicine*, edited by Alan Petersen and Robin Bunton, 94–110. London: Routledge.

Maddi, Salvatore R., and Suzanne C. Kobasa. 1984. *The hardy executive: Health under stress.* Homewood, IL: Dow Jones-Irwin.

Marshall, Barbara L. 2002. "Hard science": Gendered constructions of sexual dysfunction in the "Viagra Age." *Sexualities* 5:131–158.

Matthews, Karen A., and Suzanne G. Haynes. 1986. Type A behavior pattern and coronary disease risk: Update and critical evaluation. *American Journal of Epidemiology* 123:923–960.

McCranie, Edward W., Vickie A. Lambert, and Clinton E. Lambert, Jr. 1987. Work stress, hardiness, and burnout among hospital staff nurses. *Nursing Research* 36:374–378.

McEwen, Bruce S. 2000. The neurobiology of stress: From serendipity to clinical relevance. *Brain Research* 886:172–189.

McFarlane, Leslie. 1976. *Ghost of the Hardy boys.* New York: Methuen.

McKetney, E. C., and David R. Ragland. 1996. John Henryism, education, and blood pressure in young adults. *American Journal of Epidemiology* 143:787–791.

McKinlay, John B. 1981. From "promising report" to "standard procedure": Seven stages in the career of a medical innovation. *Milbank Memorial Fund Quarterly/Health and Society* 59(3):374–411.

McMahon, Anthony. 1993. Male readings of feminist theory: The psychologization of sexual politics in the masculinity literature. *Theory and Society* 22(5):675–696.

Merton, Robert K. 1957. *Social theory and social structure.* Glencoe, IL: Free Press.

Meryn, Siegfried, and Alejandro R. Jadad. 2001. The future of men and their health: Are men in danger of extinction? *British Medical Journal* 323:1013–1014.

Messner, Michael A. 1997. *Politics of masculinities: Men in movements.* Thousand Oaks, CA: Sage.

———. 1998. The limits of "the male sex role": An analysis of the men's liberation and men's rights movements' discourse. *Gender and Society* 12:255–276.

Meyer, Jack. 2003. Improving men's health: Developing a long-term strategy. *American Journal of Public Health* 93:709–711.

Miller, Todd Q., Charles W. Turner, R. Scott Tindale, Emil J. Posavac, and Bernard L. Dugoni. 1991. Reasons for the trend toward null findings in research on Type A behavior. *Psychological Bulletin* 19:469–485.

Mills, C. Wright. 1951. *White collar: The American middle classes.* New York: Oxford Univ. Press.

———. 1959. *The sociological imagination.* New York: Oxford Univ. Press.

Muntaner, Charles, John W. Lynch, Marianne Hillemeier, Ju Hee Lee, Richard David, Joan Benach, and Carme Borrell. 2002. Economic inequality, working-class power, social capital, and cause-specific mortality in wealthy countries. *International Journal of Health Services* 32:629–656.

Navarro, Vicente. 2002. A critique of social capital. *International Journal of Health Services* 32:423–432.

Nonn, Timothy. 1995. Renewal as retreat: The battle for men's souls. In *The politics of manhood*, edited by Michael S. Kimmel, 173–185. Philadelphia: Temple Univ. Press.

Osler, William. 1910. Angina pectoris. *Lancet* 88:839–844.

Ouelette Kobasa, Suzanne C. 1993. Inquiries into hardiness. In *Handbook of stress: Theoretical and clinical aspects*, edited by L. Goldberger and Schlomo Breznitz, 2nd ed., 77–100. New York: Free Press.

Parsons, Talcott. 1942. Age and sex in the social structure of the United States. *American Sociological Review* 7:604–616.

———. 1951. *The social system*. New York: Free Press.

———. 1979. Definitions of health and illness in the light of American values and social structure. In *Patients, physicians and illness*, edited by E. Gartly Jaco, 3rd ed., 120–144. New York: Free Press.

Parsons, Talcott, and Robert F. Bales. 1955. *Family, socialization and interaction process*. Glencoe, IL: Free Press.

Pearce, Neil, and George Davey Smith. 2003. Is social capital the key to inequalities in health? *American Journal of Public Health* 93:122–129.

Peter, Richard, and Johannes Siegrist. 1997. Chronic work stress, sickness absence, and hypertension in middle managers: General or specific sociological explanations? *Social Science and Medicine* 45:1111–1120.

Petersen, Alan. 1998. *Unmasking the masculine: Men and identity in a sceptical age*. London: Sage.

Pleck, Joseph H. 1976. The male sex role: Definitions, problems, and sources of change. *Journal of Social Issues* 32:155–164.

———. 1981. *The myth of masculinity*. Cambridge, MA: MIT Press.

Popper, Karl R. 1962. *The open society and its enemies*. Vol. 2 of *The high tide of prophecy: Hegel, Marx, and the aftermath*. 4th ed. London: Routledge & Kegan Paul.

Price, Virginia Ann. 1982. *Type A behavior pattern: A model for research and practice*. New York: Academic Press.

Prior, Lindsay. 1985. Making sense of mortality. *Sociology of Health and Illness* 7:167–190.

———. 1989. *The social organization of death: Medical discourse and social practices in Belfast*. Basingstoke, U.K.: Macmillan.

Putnam, Robert. 1995. Bowling alone: America's declining social capital. *Journal of Democracy* 6:65–78.

———. 2000. *Bowling alone: The collapse and revival of American community*. New York: Simon & Schuster.

Redfield, Margaret M. 2002. Heart failure—An epidemic of uncertain proportions. *New England Journal of Medicine* 347:1442–1444.

Reverby, Susan M., ed. 2000. *Tuskegee's truth: Rethinking the Tuskegee Syphilis Study*. Chapel Hill: Univ. of North Carolina Press.

Review Panel on Coronary-Prone Behavior and Coronary Heart Disease. 1981. Coronary-prone behavior and coronary heart disease: A critical review. *Circulation* 63:1199–1215.

Rieff, Philip. 1959. *Freud: The mind of the moralist.* New York: Viking Press.

———. 1966. *Triumph of the therapeutic: Uses of faith after Freud.* New York: Harper & Row.

Riesman, David. 1950. *The lonely crowd: A study of the changing American character.* New Haven, CT: Yale Univ. Press.

Riessman, Catherine Kohler. 1992. Women and medicalization: A new perspective. In *Inventing women: Science, technology and gender,* edited by Gill Kirkup and Laurie Smith Keller, 123–144. Milton Keynes, U.K.: Polity Press. Previously published in *Social Policy* (summer 1983): 3–19.

Riska, Elianne. 2000. The rise and fall of Type A man. *Social Science and Medicine* 51:1665–1674.

———. 2002. From Type A man to the hardy man: Masculinity and health. *Sociology of Health and Illness* 24:347–358.

———. 2003. Gendering the medicalization thesis. *Advances in Gender Research* 7:61–89.

Riska, Elianne, and Sirpa Wrede. 2003. The hardy nurse: A professional discourse on self-regulation and emotion control in a female profession. In *Conceptual and comparative studies of Continental European and Anglo-American sociology of professions,* edited by Lennart Svensson and Julia Evetts, 153–162. Göteborg, Sweden: Research Report No. 129, Department of Sociology, Göteborg Univ.

Robinson, Sally. 2000. *Marked men: White masculinity in crisis.* New York: Columbia Univ. Press.

———. 2002. Men's liberation, men's wounds: Emotion, sexuality and reconstruction of masculinity in the 1970s. In *Boys don't cry? Rethinking narratives of masculinity and emotion in the U.S.,* edited by Milette Shamir and Jennifer Travis, 205–229. New York: Columbia Univ. Press.

Rose, Nikolas. 1997. Assembling the modern self. In *Rewriting the self: Histories from the Renaissance to the present,* edited by Roy Porter, 224–248. London: Routledge.

———. 1999. *Governing the soul: The shaping of the private self.* 2nd ed. London: Free Association Books.

Rose, Stephen M. 1972. *The betrayal of the poor: The transformation of community action.* Cambridge, MA: Schenkman Publishing Company.

Rosenfield, Sarah. 1992. The cost of sharing: Wives' employment and husbands' mental health. *Journal of Health and Social Behavior* 33:213–225.

Rosenman, Ray H. 1978. The interview method of assessment of coronary-prone behavior pattern. In *Coronary-prone behavior,* edited by Theodore M. Dembroski, Stephen M. Weiss, Jim L. Shields, Suzane L. Haynes, and Feinleib Manning, 55–69. New York: Springer-Verlag.

Rosenman, Ray H., and Meyer Friedman. 1971. The central nervous system and coronary heart disease. *Hospital Practice* 6 (October): 87–97.

Rosenman, Ray H., Meyer Friedman, Reuben Straus et al. 1970. Coronary heart disease in the Western Collaborative Group Study: A follow-up experience of 4½ years. *Journal of Chronic Disease* 23:173–190.

Rosenman, Ray H., Richard J. Brand, C. David Jenkins, Meyer Friedman, Reuben Straus, and Moses Wurm. 1975. Coronary heart disease in the Western Collaborative Group Study: Follow-up experience of 8½ years. *Journal of the American Medical Association* 233:872–877.

Roskies, Ethel. 1987. *Stress management for the healthy Type A: Theory and practice.* New York: Guilford Press.

Ross, Catherine E., and John Mirowsky. 2001. Neighborhood disadvantage, disorder, and health. *Journal of Health and Social Behavior* 42:258–276.

Rothman, Barbara Katz. 1998. *Genetic maps and human imaginations: The limits of science in understanding who we are.* New York: W.W. Norton & Company.

Ruzek, Sheryl Burt. 1978. *The women's health movement: Feminist alternatives to medical control.* New York: Praeger.

Sabo, Donald. 2000. Men's health studies: Origins and trends. *Journal of American College Health* 49:133–142.

Sabo, Donald, and David Frederick Gordon. 1995. Rethinking men's health and illness: The relevance of gender studies. In *Men's health and illness: Gender, power and the body*, edited by Donald Sabo and David Frederick Gordon, 1–21. Thousand Oaks, CA: Sage.

Sapolsky, Robert M. 1994. *Why zebras don't get ulcers: A guide to stress, stress-related diseases and coping.* New York: N. H. Freeman & Company.

Sardell, Alice. 1988. *The U.S. experiment in social medicine: The Community Health Center Program, 1965–1986.* Pittsburg, PA: Univ. of Pittsburg Press.

Schmied, Lori A., and Kathleen A. Lawler. 1986. Hardiness, Type A behavior and the stress-illness relation in working women. *Journal of Personality and Social Psychology* 51:1218–1223.

Schofield, Toni, R. W. Connell, Linley Walker, Julian F. Wood, and Dianne L. Butland. 2000. Understanding men's health and illness: A gender-relations approach to policy, research, and practice. *Journal of American College Health* 48:247–256.

Sennett, Richard. 1998. *The corrosion of character: The personal consequences of work in the new capitalism.* New York: W.W. Norton & Company.

Shim, Janet K. 2002. Understanding the routinised inclusion of race, socioeconomic status and sex in epidemiology: The utility of concepts from technoscience studies. *Sociology of Health and Illness* 24:129–150.

Simoni, Patricia S., and John J. Paterson. 1997. Hardiness, coping, and burnout in the nursing workplace. *Journal of Professional Nursing* 13:178–185.

Staples, Robert. 1982. *Black masculinity: The black male's role in American society.* San Francisco: The Black Scholar Press.

———. 1995a. Stereotypes of black male sexuality: The facts behind the myths. In *Men's lives*, edited by Michael S. Kimmel and Michael A. Messner, 3rd ed., 375–380. Boston: Allyn & Bacon.

———. 1995b. Health among African-American males. In *Men's health and illness: Gender, power, and the body*, edited by David Sabo and David Frederick Gordon, 121–138. Thousand Oaks, CA: Sage.

Stolley, Paul D. 1999. Race in epidemiology. *International Journal of Health Services* 29:905–909.

Stone, Stephanie V., and Paul T. Costa. 1990. Disease-prone or distress-prone personality? The role of neuroticism in coronary heart disease. In *Personality and disease*, edited by Howard S. Friedman, 178–200. New York: John Wiley.

Sundquist, Jan, and Marilyn A. Winkleby. 1999. Cardiovascular risk factors in Mexican American adults: A transcultural analysis of NHANES III, 1988–1994. *American Journal of Public Health* 89:723–730.

Susman, Warren I. 1984. *Culture as history: The transformation of American society in the twentieth century.* New York: Pantheon Books.

Temoshok, Lydia. 1987. Personality, coping style, emotion and cancer: Towards an integrative model. *Cancer Surveys* 6:545–567.

Temoshok, Lydia, Bruce W. Heller, Richard W. Sagebiel, Mardsen S. Blois, David M. Sweet, Ralph J. DiClemente, and Marc L. Gold. 1985. The relationship of psychosocial factors to prognostic indicators in cutaneous malignant melanoma. *Journal of Psychosomatic Research* 29:139–153.

Theriot, Nancy M. 1993. Women's voices in nineteenth century medical discourse: A step toward deconstructing science. *Signs* 19:1–31.

Timmermans, Stefan, and Marc Berg. 2003. The practice of medical technology. *Sociology of Health and Illness* 25:97–114.

Tocqueville, Alexis de. 1945. *Democracy in America.* Vol. 2. New York: Random House/Vintage.

Treadwell, Henrie, and Marguerite Ro. 2003. Poverty, race, and the invisible men. *American Journal of Public Health* 93:705–706.

U.S. National Center for Health Statistics. 2003. *Health, United States 2002,* www.cdc.gov/nchs (table 37).

U.S. National Library of Medicine. 1998. *Medical subject headings: Annotated alphabetic list.* Bethesda, MD: National Institutes of Health.

———. 2003. Medline: PubMed, www.ncbi.nlm.nih.gov.pubmed (accessed December 23, 2003).

Wagner, David. 1997. *The new temperance: The American obsession with sin and vice.* Boulder, CO: Westview Press.

Wainwright, David, and Michael Calnan. 2002. *Work stress: The making of a modern epidemic.* Buckingham, U.K.: Open Univ. Press.

Waitzkin, Howard. 2000. *The second sickness: Contradictions of capitalist health care.* Rev. ed. Lanham, MD: Rowman & Littlefield.

Walby, Sylvia. 1990. *Theorizing patriarchy.* Oxford: Basil Blackwell.

Waldron, Ingrid. 1995. Contributions of changing gender differences in behavior and social roles to changing differences in mortality. In *Men's health and illness: Gender, power, and the body*, edited by Donald Sabo and David Frederick Gordon, 22–45. Thousand Oaks, CA: Sage.

Weber, Max. 1958. *The Protestant ethic and the spirit of capitalism.* New York: Charles Scribner's Sons.

Weinrich, Sally P., Martin C. Weinrich, Julian E. Keil, Peter C. Gates, and Ellen Potter. 1988. The John Henryism and Framingham Type A scales: Measurement properties in elderly blacks and whites. *American Journal of Epidemiology* 128:165–178.

Weiss, Stephen M., Susan M. Czajkowski, Sally A. Shumaker, and Roger T. Anderson. 1990. Psychosocial factors in coronary heart disease. In *Preventive aspects of coronary heart disease,* edited by Edward D. Frohlich, 135–148. Philadelphia: F. A. Davis Company.

Welch, Norman A. 1964. Unity in medicine (presidential inaugural address). *Journal of American Medical Association* 189:223–225.

White, Alan, and Lesley Lockyer. 2001. Tackling coronary heart disease: A gender sensitive approach needed. *British Medical Journal* 323:1016–1017.

Whitehead, Steven M. 2002. *Men and masculinities.* Cambridge, U.K.: Polity Press.

Wiebe, Deborah J., and Debra Moehle McCallum. 1986. Health practices and hardiness as mediators in the stress-illness relationship. *Health Psychology* 5:425–438.

Wiist, William H., and John M. Flack. 1992. A test of the John Henryism hypothesis: Cholesterol and blood pressure. *Journal of Behavioral Medicine* 15:15–29.

Wilkinson, Richard G. 1996. *Unhealthy societies: The affliction of inequality.* London: Routledge.

Williams, David R. 2003. The health of men: Structured inequalities and opportunities. *American Journal of Public Health* 93:724–731.

Williams, David R., Harold W. Neighbors, and James S. Jackson. 2003. Racial/ethnic discrimination and health: Findings from community studies. *American Journal of Public Health* 93:200–208.

Williams, Simon J. 1998. "Capitalising" on emotions? Rethinking the inequalities in health debate. *Sociology* 32:121–139.

Williams, Simon J., and Gillian Bendelow. 1998. *The lived body: Sociological themes, embodied issues.* London: Routledge.

Winant, Howard. 2000. Race and race theory. *Annual Review of Sociology* 26:169–185.

Young, Allan. 1980. The discourse on stress and the reproduction of conventional knowledge. *Social Science and Medicine* 14B, 133–146.

Zborowski, Marc. 1952. Cultural components in response to pain. *Journal of Social Issues* 8:16–30.

Zola, Irving K. 1966. Culture and symptoms: An analysis of patients presenting complaints. *American Sociological Review* 31:615–631.

———. 1972. Medicine as an institution of social control. *Sociological Review* 20:487–504.

Index

Sabo, Donald, 14, 127
Sapolsky, Robert M., 53, 111, 122
Sardell, Alice, 74
Scandinavia, 87
Schmied, Lori A., 37
Schofield, Toni, 3, 15–17, 127
scientific discovery, 23, 31, 88, 96–99
scientific racism. *See* race
script, 12, 37–38, 48, 56, 82, 97
self: disciplined self, 7–8, 22, 65, 71,
    106, 114; embodied self, 2, 28;
    grammar of the self, 50, 57, 118;
    inner self, 18, 30, 49, 83, 107, 109,
    112; moral self, 25, 57, 80, 113,
    118; pathologized, 18–19, 112;
    reflexive self, 21; regulation of the
    self, 7, 83, 106–7; technologies of
    the self, 7–8, 22, 63, 106;
    victimized, 5, 11–12, 109; wounded,
    16, 18, 109, 112
self-control, 22, 29, 54, 65–66, 70–71,
    83, 106–8, 112, 115
self-made man, 4–5, 29, 39, 66
Sennett, Richard, 7, 64, 105, 108
sex-role theory, 2, 13, 17, 19, 97, 102–3,
    110, 112–14, 127; critique of, 13, 17;
    healthy sex role identity, 13, 63, 71,
    109, 113; modern male sex role, 14,
    60, 105; sex-role-identity
    perspective, 13–14, 114; sex-role-
    strain perspective, 14, 22; traditional
    male sex role, 14, 30–31, 105–6, 110
Shim, Janet K., 98
sick-role theory, 20
Simoni, Patricia S., 64
social behavior, 19, 24, 43, 65, 102,
    104, 127
social capital, 108–9, 123–26
social class, 4, 15, 30, 44, 49, 55, 57,
    66, 68, 81, 86; middle class, 1–5, 7,
    19, 24–25, 30–32, 37–38, 44–45, 50,
    54–56, 59–60, 64–66, 68, 71, 74,
    76–77, 80, 82–84, 95, 104, 109–12,
    114–15, 117–19, 124; working class,
    79, 90, 104, 117

social constructionist perspective, 8, 23,
    85, 89, 112
social movement, 5; men's movement,
    13–15; women's movement, 5, 13,
    19, 22
social order, 2, 8, 21, 24, 41, 50, 101,
    103–5, 110–11, 113, 126–27;
    economic order, 21, 99, 104–5, 109,
    113, 117, 126; gender order, 2, 7, 16,
    18, 22, 41, 65, 70, 104, 110, 115,
    120, 127; racial order, 2, 8, 25, 50,
    82, 89, 104
social ritualism, 102, 107
social structure, 2, 8, 21, 37, 49–50, 54,
    70, 87, 101–3, 109
socialization, 62–63, 110
sociological determinism. *See*
    determinism
space of anxiety, 8
space of configuration, 29
Staples, Robert, 3, 82
Stolley, Paul D., 81
Stone, Stephanie V., 53
Stratemeyer, Edward, 67
stress, 6, 8, 28, 31–32, 42–43, 45, 47,
    59–65, 70–71, 85, 96, 111, 116,
    120–22, 125–26
stressors, 40, 42, 53, 78, 84, 111
Structured Interview. *See* methodology
Sundquist, Jan, 81
surveillance medicine, 27–28, 86–87
Susman, Warren I., 24, 50, 69

technologies of the self, 7–8, 22, 63,
    106
Temoshok, Lydia, 40–41
Theriot, Nancy M., 22
Timmermans, Stefan, 22
Tocqueville, Alexis de, 27
Treadwell, Henrie, 3
Type A. *See* personality
Type A Behavioral Pattern (TABP), 6,
    28, 35–36, 48, 51, 54, 91, 96, 117.
    See also Type A
Type B. *See* personality

About the Author

Elianne Riska is Professor of Sociology in the Swedish School of Social Science at the University of Helsinki, Finland. She was the von Willebrand-Fahlbeck Professor of Sociology and Statistics at Åbo Akademi University, Åbo, Finland, from 1985 to 2004. She received her Ph.D. in sociology from the State University of New York, Stony Brook, in 1974 and was an assistant and associate professor of sociology in the Department of Sociology and College of Human Medicine at Michigan State University from 1974 to 1981. Her most recent books include *Gender, Work and Medicine* (Sage 1993), *Gendered Moods* (Routledge 1995), and *Medical Careers and Feminist Agendas: American, Scandinavian, and Russian Women Physicians* (Aldine de Gruyter 2001).